Reiki and Chakras

Unlocking the Secrets of Aura Cleansing and Reiki Self-healing

(Learning Reiki Symbols and Acquiring Tips for Reiki Meditation and Reiki Psychic Unlocking Your Chakras)

Raven Petter

Published by Rob Miles

Raven Petter

All Rights Reserved

Reiki and Chakras: Unlocking the Secrets of Aura Cleansing and Reiki Self-healing (Learning Reiki Symbols and Acquiring Tips for Reiki Meditation and Reiki Psychic Unlocking Your Chakras)

ISBN 978-1-989990-53-7

All rights reserved. No part of this guide may be reproduced in any form without permission in writing from the publisher except in the case of brief quotations embodied in critical articles or reviews.

Legal & Disclaimer

The information contained in this book is not designed to replace or take the place of any form of medicine or professional medical advice. The information in this book has been provided for educational and entertainment purposes only.

The information contained in this book has been compiled from sources deemed reliable, and it is accurate to the best of the Author's knowledge; however, the Author cannot guarantee its accuracy and validity and cannot be held liable for any errors or omissions. Changes are periodically made to this book. You must consult your doctor or get professional medical advice before using any of the suggested remedies, techniques, or information in this book.

Upon using the information contained in this book, you agree to hold harmless the Author from and against any damages, costs, and expenses, including any legal fees potentially resulting from the application of any of the information provided by this guide. This disclaimer applies to any damages or injury caused by the use and application, whether directly or indirectly, of any advice or information presented, whether for breach of contract, tort, negligence, personal injury, criminal intent, or under any other cause of action.

You agree to accept all risks of using the information presented inside this book. You need to consult a professional medical practitioner in order to ensure you are both able and healthy enough to participate in this program.

Table of Contents

INTRODUCTION 1

CHAPTER 1: WHERE YOGA COMES FROM 2

CHAPTER 2: DIFFERENT REIKI LEVELS 8

CHAPTER 3: LEARNING ABOUT REIKI 19

CHAPTER 4: IS REIKI VITALITY TORMENT ALLEVIATION GENUINE? 22

CHAPTER 5: LEARN REIKI HEALING IN 30 MINUTES OR LESS 26

CHAPTER 6: A VIEW OF THE USUI STORY 51

CHAPTER 7: WHAT BEING A REIKI TEACHER / ATTUNER INVOLVES 65

CHAPTER 8: WHAT ARE THE FIVE PRECEPTS? 74

CHAPTER 9: FIFTEEN REASONS TO APPLY REIKI TO YOUR OWN LIFE 88

CHAPTER 10: TAOIST SYSTEM OF THE FIVE PHASES OF THE CHI CYCLE 96

- CHAPTER 11: THE SOLAR PLEXUS CHAKRA 106
- CHAPTER 12: CHAKRAS – THE ENERGY CENTRES 112
- CHAPTER 13: AURA/ MAGNETIC FIELD 133
- CHAPTER 14: THE SIXTH CHAKRA 142
- CHAPTER 15: MEDITATION 146
- CHAPTER 16: TIMEOUT: HOW TO PERFORM A QUICK HEALING SESSION.. 151
- CHAPTER 17: CHAKRAS AND AURA................................ 163
- CHAPTER 18: THE HISTORY OF REIKI.............................. 177
- CHAPTER 19: RECEIVING ANGELIC REIKI 191
- CHAPTER 20: WHAT MAKES A GOOD HEALER?.............. 195
- CONCLUSION.. 201

Introduction

Reiki is a vital and a fundamental part of Japanese tradition. It is a Japanese technique which has been and is mainly used to reduce stress, induce relaxation and promote healing. It is carried out by "laying on hands" and is solely based on the concept that the unseen life force energy flows through the body and is responsible for keeping us alive and healthy. If your life force energy is weak, your body will become more prone to illnesses and you will be more likely to be easily stressed out. On the other hand, if it is high, you will be more capable of being healthy and, best of all, happy.

Chapter 1: Where Yoga Comes From

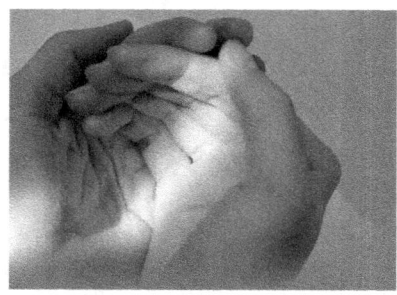

The above quotation tells you about what yoga is from the stance of someone who practices it on a regular basis. The practice of yoga goes back to India and you may be surprised that its practice began as early as around the time of 500 B.C.E. It was practiced as a means to get closer to enlightenment by the Brahman people and, at that time, involved chants, different rituals and mantras. We know today that mantras are still used by some yoga practitioners, and to simplify what these are, I would explain that they are words that the mind concentrates on while practicing yoga, in order to keep the mind occupied and focused so that trains of thought do not get in the way of the yoga practice. That's simplifying it a little, but I have done that intentionally, since you are looking into starting yoga and to explain it in any more complex a way may scare you off. That's not my intention.

Classical yoga followed and this included many of the rituals that people follow in today's yoga practice including following a path to lead you to enlightenment. The Buddhist monks practice this in their own rituals but for the layman, what you gain from your everyday practice of yoga in a modern world is very similar. You reach a moment where you suddenly realize the power of the mind and the limitlessness of it that you cannot discover by any other means. Yoga meditation branches off from this classical yoga and although you don't need to know all of the technical data on this, you will learn in the following chapters how meditation helps to lead you to an enlightened state and that is what gives you inner joy. That's what we seek when we practice meditation and it can indeed make you very happy and contented indeed.

Tantra yoga, or pre classical yoga is a little more touchy feely and is perhaps not what you are looking for and this included helping the healing process, though this can also be done by using Hatha yoga which is more in line with modern day yoga practice. The more apt you get at yoga practice, the more your muscles and tendons are able to stretch and the energy that goes through your body is able to avoid blockages. These blockages may be caused by any number of things from mental problems right through the spectrum to problems with posture.

Today's yoga

Today's yoga, as imported to the West, is a combination of all the different types of yoga and I believe has been developed in a way that fits in with modern western society and the way that people live their lives. It can be done in sessions and then taken to the privacy of your own home and although our backgrounds are very different from the different religious groups who practice yoga in India and other countries, we are able to relate to it, since its teaching is logical. As a learner, you are walked through the stages that begin to piece it all together and help you to make sense of it.

The things that you will learn include breathing techniques to help oxygen flow within the body. Relaxation techniques – to stave off the harsh pressures of today's world, and meditation techniques – to hone in on your inner needs. You may think that it all sounds very idealistic, but it has been proven over thousands of years to be beneficial. I write from a Buddhist stance and believe that yoga and yoga meditation makes you more aware of other people and your place among them. It also builds confidence, enables you to gain self-esteem and teaches you how to deal with things such as stress, so that they no longer impede your life.

Now that you know where yoga comes from, it's time to move onto our introduction as this is important. Without the introductory stages, you will often find that you will fail and it is for this reason that they have been given so much emphasis. You have to think of the way that your mind works, the way that you breathe and the way that you use that breath to make you stronger and more spiritually aware. This, in turn, can make you a lot happier and open up the channels of energy that run through every human being. You may have heard about acupuncture and may even know about the energy points that make up the qi and chee, or balance of energies. In yoga, you have much the same thing, though in this case, they have called it something else. Chakras are the areas in the body which allow energy to pass and yoga will help you to free up these areas so that your bodily balance and wellbeing are catered for in a very full and all-encompassing manner.

Remember, as you go through the process of learning, it is never about how quickly you perform the exercises. This isn't a sport. It's about how thoroughly you have absorbed the lesson and are able to practice it. It is better therefore to take things slowly – at your own pace – and learn slowly and methodically, rather than to go into it too quickly and glean bad habits from the commencement.

Chapter 2: Different Reiki Levels

There are four stages of Reiki but normally, Reiki 3 and Reiki 4 are always combined as one. Essentially, Reiki 1 is use for healing one's self while Reiki 2 is used to heal other people. Reiki 3, also referred to as Reiki Master, is used to give attunements to other people while Reiki 4 is used to teach Reiki healing to those who want to learn.

There are a lot of Reiki Masters who can give you attunements for Reiki 1, 2, and 3 within a brief period of time. You can actually receive your attunement over one weekend. But it is also possible to receive an "absent attunement" from a Reiki Master who has been trained in it.

The giving of an attunement is normally considered a precious gift not only for the person receiving it, but also for the Reiki

Master giving it. During the attunement process, no energy is detracted from the giver or the Reiki Master but the receiver will be given the benefit of attunement for the rest of his or her life.

Reiki 1

Reiki 1 is considered as the stage where a Reiki healer can give healing to his or her own self when practicing healing with other people such as loved ones and friends. At this stage, a Reiki healer is discouraged from charging fees for the Reiki healing that they perform on other people and should not yet promote their healing service to others. As a Reiki 1 healer, you will still be learning how to channel or control the healing energies of Reiki in an effective manner. Use this stage to learn more about yourself and how you can become an effective Reiki healer.

Almost anyone can be attuned to Reiki 1 healing, as long as they ask for it and are willing to learn the practice. When you become attuned, you will be opened to the Divine energies, whether you choose to intentionally or unintentionally use those energies to heal yourself or other people. Many people stop performing Reiki healing after a brief time and only a few choose to continue performing Reiki healing and progressing to more advanced levels.

When you have been attuned to Reiki 1 healing, you should make the most out of it, not only by healing yourself but also by discovering more about yourself. More often than not, people seek to learn Reiki when they experience issues in their lives that need to be attended to and be healed. Some of these issues may be healed within a short period of time but some issues may be more serious and may require a longer period of time to completely heal.

But when you are in Reiki 1, you do not really need to be perfect and healed in all manners before you can proceed to the second Reiki level. But you will definitely need to be willing and committed to take a journey within yourself and discover more about yourself before you can continue with Reiki healing with other people. It is possible that your soul may have very minimal imbalance, which will only need minimal self-healing. This means that your stay in the first Reiki level may be short.

Once you've learned about it and heal yourself with Reiki energy, you will gain insight into the workings of your own soul and into the physical, emotional, mental, and physical facets of your being. This will then lead you to better understand and heal other people.

Normally, those aspects of yourself that you write off as a "no problem" area are frequently the areas that require the most healing and attention. People normally hide their deepest and darkest fears into the areas they insist do not need any attention. When you have been attuned with Reiki 1 healing and when you are determined to heal yourself, the issues and problems that require healing will come to light so you can heal them and be ultimately free from them. A lot of people overlook the importance of this process and they request to be attuned to Reiki 2 level without truly seeing their inner fears and pain that require healing. Don't make the same mistake and embrace this journey as an important part of your personal growth.

Some people believe that it is Reiki itself that selects the people who will be bestowed with its energy, instead of the other way around. But I think that this is not completely true. As long as you have trust and belief in the power of Reiki and how effective it is as a healing method and a spiritual path toward freedom, you can trust and believe in the immeasurable divine guidance you can achieve from it. All of us are gifted with free will. There are a lot of Reiki healers and Reiki Masters who went into learning about Reiki and becoming attuned even when they have not received any sacred sign that it is the right thing for them to do. All of us are spiritual beings within our human forms. Therefore, it is wise and but natural for us to deliberately undertake things that can bring us both personal and spiritual growth.

But this is not to say that Reiki is the best path for everyone. There are people who have been given attunements by Reiki Masters they know and those people were not able to completely embrace the practice because they were not interested. There have been a lot of indications that show that Reiki is an effective healing system for some people but not for everyone. People who seek to be healed and to gain spiritual insight about their own selves will be directed toward the right path. The Reiki Masters are available to provide guidance to help each of us to know what is best for us through the Reiki Master's own wisdom and through divine guidance.

For many people, their training and initiation to the first level of Reiki healing is both a wonderful experience to discover not only the power of Reiki but their own spirituality, as well. It can help you to see a completely new world that can make you feel liberated, empowered, and totally wonderful. A lot of people are actually tempted to proceed with the second level of Reiki just to be able to experience these wonderful feelings at a more intense degree. It is quite easy to consider Reiki as the complete answer and that it can restore your health and empower you without much effort from your end. You need to realize that Reiki is not your ticket to acquire your dream life but it can definitely be your ticket for an extraordinary journey that can lead you toward your dreams.

Reiki 2

At the second Reiki level, you will receive another attunement, which will significantly increase your healing power. As a Reiki 2 healer, you may already promote yourself as a Reiki healer and begin charging other people for your healing services, if you wish. At this level, you have a lot more flexibility in the practice of Reiki healing and you can start sending Reiki energy into different areas that require healing, which can even include the past or the future of the person you are healing. You will also be expected to learn how to employ the Reiki energies in all aspects of your life and how to utilize the sacred Reiki symbols into your healing practice.

Before being initiated into Reiki, your Reiki Master may ask you if you have made a sincere effort in completely healing yourself and in controlling the Reiki energies that flow within you. You need to show that you have achieved a sufficient level of spiritual insight about yourself. You may also be required to have practiced Reiki healing on your own loved ones and friends. You need to be able to show that you have completely embraced Reiki energies as an effective healing system. You will need to demonstrate your honest intention of using Reiki to heal other people through your own love and compassion for mankind.

Reiki 3 (Reiki Master) and Reiki 4 (Reiki Teacher)

When you have been attuned as Reiki 3 or Reiki Master, you will already be able to give attunement to other Reiki healers who are at levels 1 to 3. On the other hand, if you are a Reiki 4 or a Reiki Teacher, you are required to be competent enough to teach Reiki to other people. Normally, attunement to Reiki 3 and Reiki 4 levels are performed at the same time. Some Reiki Masters who are also Reiki Teachers prefer to call themselves as just a Reiki Master whereas others prefer to be called Reiki Master/Teacher to show the difference between level 3 and level 4.

To be given attunement as a Reiki Master, you would have demonstrated your full commitment, not only to your own spiritual growth and development but also to other people's. When you are given the Reiki Master attunement, your life will definitely be changed permanently. People who have been given attunement to Reiki 1 may choose to continue their Reiki practice or not but this should not be the same case for a Reiki Master. When you choose to become initiated as a Reiki Master, it comes with your affirmation that you wish to become one of the leaders in the Reiki healing practice.

A true Reiki Master affirms, in spirit, that he wants to become one of the ambassadors of great love in this world. You should only ask for a Reiki Master attunement after you have performed a careful deliberation of how it will affect the rest of your life. You need to accept the Reiki Master attunement with a great sense of respect for and dedication to the healing system of Reiki.

Chapter 3: Learning About Reiki

Synopsis

Though reiki has been around for some time, it is only in recent times it is slowly becoming a viable alternative to seeking conventional medical treatments. Learning or acquiring this art form does not require extensive intellectual capacities, nor does it require years of study to master. The beauty of reiki is that it is so accessible that the tenants can be passed on from teacher to student without much discrimination.

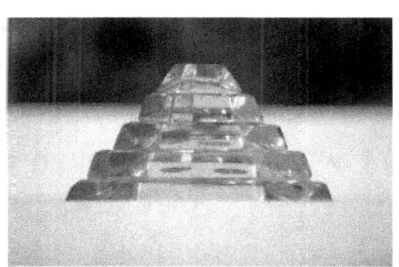

Getting Schooled

Achieving the purest and clearest mind set is the basis of reiki because the energy needed to make a successful transfer to another individual for healing purposes consists of positive energy. Some people even connect this to being one with body and mind which yet some others say has a certain connection directly to God.

Some people who have taken this art form very seriously attest to having psychic sensitivity. Some even claim to have the "third eye" capabilities, increased awareness of the surroundings even to its molecular levels.

All these serve practically when addressing one's general health issues. The ability to harness this positive energy translates to the ability to heal and be healed. People who don't want to go through extensive western style medical processes sometimes find miraculous results when reiki is practiced. Reiki is an element that once learnt and mastered stays with the individual for life. It is not something that can be forgotten easily.

The successful practice of reiki affects the body, mind, and emotions. As toxins that are stored in the body system over time are often attributed to causing much negativity in the body, practicing reiki enables the release process to begin, using positive energy. Understanding the seriousness of negative energy impacts, enables reiki to be an effective means of gaining optimum health conditions. However to successfully practice reiki, one has to be prepared to make certain lifestyle changes. These requirements all have beneficial qualities.

Chapter 4: Is Reiki vitality torment alleviation genuine?

Amid my time working in a nursing home, I went through numerous hours with patients who needed to pick between anguishing agonies or a medication actuated trance. Around then, the force of mending touch or Reiki vitality recuperating treatment was not perceived or acknowledged. Acting from a longing to help, medical attendants and hospice laborers have taken it upon themselves to take in the recuperating craftsmanship and add it to their treatment choices.

In the wake of getting Reiki vitality recuperating treatment from a hospice attendant, he was taught to utilize Reiki vitality. He was taught about building his "purpose" to utilize Reiki vitality, something that appears to be essential, with the end goal Reiki should be compelling.

With Reiki and his plan, his personal satisfaction made strides. His level of solace moved forward. He found himself able to live "well with his disease". Nobody is stating that Reiki "cured" his tumor", however it did soothe his indications and the nature of his remaining days was moved forward.

In instances of cutting edge tumor, as indicated by the analyst (M. Bullock), the general patterns seen with Reiki vitality mending treatment incorporate times of adjustment, help from agony, tension, swelling and a "quiet and cool passing if demise is approaching". The creator suggests Reiki vitality recuperating treatment as a profitable compliment to be utilized by the individuals who function as a part of a hospice domain or are supporting patients in their "end-of-life voyage".

Is Reiki vitality torment help simply a placebo impact?

Analysts say "no". In the Journal of Complementary Medicine, specialists distributed the consequences of a study in which the outcomes and reactions of customers were contrasted with their starting desires. The hypothesis is that if Reiki vitality torment help were basically a placebo impact, just those patients that normal alleviation would report achievement.

Furthermore scientists measured the level of antibodies in persistent's salivation previously, then after the fact treatment. The greater part of the outcomes were contrasted with a control amass that got no treatment.

Specialists found that the rate of patients who reported alleviation of agony was much higher than would regularly be normal from a placebo impact. 14% is a typical rate for placebo incited agony alleviation. 55% was the rate of customers in the study who reported that Reiki vitality torment alleviation was successful. Positive reactions did not give off an impression of being identified with the customer's beginning desires or convictions.

Moreover, the customers who were dealt with by the most experienced Reiki specialists had essentially more elevated amounts of antibodies in their spit. The scientists presumed that the treatment adequately diminished push and agony, while enhancing the body's capacity to battle of disease and that the discoveries were not solely an aftereffect of the placebo impact.

Chapter 5: Learn Reiki Healing in 30 Minutes or Less

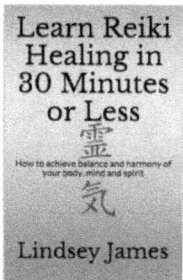

How to achieve balance and harmony of your body, mind and spirit

INTRODUCTION TO REIKI HEALING

Reiki, Japanese for universal life force energy, is a healing technique that that heals on every level; mental, physical, spiritual and emotional, by utilizing the universal life force, the energy that pervades throughout the whole universe and every living thing.

In China, this force is known as chi or qi, in India, prana, and in Japan, ki. From this, the name reiki is derived. This force flows freely throughout our bodies and into an energy field encompassing them.

This energy controls every bodily process on every level; emotional, mental and physical. So long as this energy flows harmoniously, good heath prevails. However, imbalances in the flow result in physical and mental illnesses.

In reiki healing treatments, universal life energy is channeled through the practitioner's hands and into the ailing person's body in order to balance the recipient's energy flow.

The body is not a machine constructed from isolated parts that can be fixed individually. It is a complex system, harnessing a fantastic network of energy. For true health to be restored, every aspect of our being needs to be addressed. Reiki is devoted to healing the complete person.

Reiki operates on four levels:

<u>Physical level</u>: At this level, reiki aids in pain relief, synchronizes and balances organ and gland functions and promotes a stronger immune system. It also restores chakra balance and opens blocked energy pathways. Regular treatments rid the body of toxins and maintain well-being and good heath.

<u>Emotional level</u>: On this level, reiki reduces stress and increases relaxation, which makes for stronger immunity and lasting health. Reiki eliminates energy blockages and brings suppressed emotions to the surface, which eases feelings of depression.

Mental level: Through reiki, higher levels of clarity are achieved and conquering obstacles in order to achieve goals becomes easier. Overall, you gain more self-confidence and your viewpoint on life becomes more positive.

Spiritual level: Reiki provides the ability to reach within yourself and obtain a stronger connection with your higher being. Additionally, it heightens intuition, helps in meditation and offers unlimited spiritual growth.

Although reiki is extremely powerful, it is also very simple to use as it requires no special ability or prior experience and anyone can learn it.

Reiki offers endless advantages and lets you actively participate in your own well-being. It can also help to accelerate all levels of personal growth.

BENEFITS OF REIKI HEALING

Reiki is a non-invasive healing touch therapy that helps boost mental, physical and emotional health. It also helps enhance spiritual wellbeing.

Stress reduction is one of the greatest benefits. Typically, people are better able to cope with stress and tension when they are in a relaxed state of mind. Stress has been linked to various ailments such as high blood pressure, heart disease, stroke and cancer. When the body is relaxed, the immune system triggers natural healing abilities.

Another health benefit of reiki is mental and emotional balance that helps enhance memory and improve the ability to focus. It also helps increase mental clarity. Regular treatments can help improve the mind by making it sharper and clearer.

Reiki can also help ease feelings of anger, fear and frustration and help strengthen mental health. Inner peace and harmony are excellent tools for spiritual growth. People claim to feel better and say they enjoy better sleep after experiencing touch therapy.

It has been proven that reiki can strengthen personal relationships by enhancing the ability to love and understand loved ones. It increases the level of empathy and helps create a deeper connection that allows people to bond on a deeper level, which helps relationships to grow stronger.

During therapy sessions, emotions are cleared and are prevented from draining on the mind. It promotes positive energy and aids in the reduction of anxiety and depression. It can also help decrease mood swings.

Another health benefit is the lessening of pain. People, who undergo touch therapy claim to feel less pain in various areas of the body such as the shoulders, arms, legs and back. Reiki also helps relieve pain from a variety of ailments such as arthritis, headaches and migraines.

It can also decrease inflammation in the joints and ease fatigue and asthma symptoms. Moreover, it can speed-up recovery from a long term illness or from surgery and can reduce the side effects of certain medications used during recovery.

Reiki is fast becoming an accepted practice in hospitals and clinics and is one of the most effective and best therapeutic methods available to help improve overall physical and mental health.

HISTORY OF REIKI HEALING

The history of reiki begins in ancient Japan. While there are different stories it is generally accepted that the reiki can be traced back to Dr. Mikao Usui who lived in Japan in the late 1800s.

Dr Mikao Usui is said to have traveled to many different parts of the world during his life. At one point he became a Tendi Buddhist Monk. It is during this time in his life that he became enlightened to the knowledge of spiritual healing.

As Dr. Usui had traveled before becoming a monk it is believed that some outside influences were incorporated in his healing. Other forms of spiritual and physical healing such as Chinese medicine, eastern healing systems like Chi Gong and the Japanese equivalent Kiko can be found in what we today call reiki.

Dr Usui is reported to have been a very skilled healer and teacher whose fame spread very quickly throughout Japan. He opened his first clinic/school in Tokyo in 1922. The teachings and techniques that were contained in his spiritual healing system worked well for a variety of ailments. Although his school was for spiritual teaching many people were given cheap or free treatment. Usui Sensei's teachings were divided into 6 levels.

The first level was Shoden (student) which has 4 different levels. This level is where the students worked hard to increase their own spirituality. Only when this was mastered could they move to the next level of Okuden or inner teachings. It is reported that not many of his students passed this level to the next.

The last level is Shinpi-Den or mystery/secret teachings. Dr Usui was reported to have taught over 2000 people. One of these students was Chujiro Hayashi.

Dr Chujiro Hayashi is believed to be one of the few who became a master under Dr Usui. He is said to be the originator of the hand position system used in the west today. Dr Hayashi used 7 to 8 hand positions to treat the upper body. The belief that the head and torso was treating the major centers energy which would flow to the rest of the body. He may have adapted further hand positions we see used in reiki today.

It was during his time as a practitioner in Japan that Dr. Hayashi had a patient by the name of Mrs. Takada who had traveled from Hawaii. Mrs. Takada was so impressed with her healing that she became a student of Dr. Hayashi. and when she returned to Hawaii she established reiki teaching there.

Mrs. Takada was initiated to reiki master in 1938 and went on to initiate a further 22 masters.

REIKI ENERGY

The word reiki comes from two Japanese words; rei and ki.

Rei is the higher intelligence that guides the evolution of the universe and all it contains. It can help us to understand more about the universe and the world around us.

Ki is the non physical energy that is contained in all living things, not just people but also animals and plants. If a person has a high amount of ki energy they are strong and able to accept challenges that they can take on with confidence. When a person has a ki that is low they are more susceptible to illness.

A person can improve their ki level by completing breathing exercises, getting plenty of sunshine, and even getting enough sleep.

When rei and ki are put together, reiki can be thought of as an energy source that is not physical but has great healing potential using the energy sources of life guided by a spiritual power.

Reiki cannot be forced, we must find a place where we can concentrate on our energy forces and healing power without being distracted. Using reiki we can bring our minds to a healthy state, when the mind is healed the body can begin to heal.

Negative energy can exist in both the body and the mind. Practicing reiki helps the body regain its natural balance. Even negative and unhappy thoughts are harmful to the body and they, along with any toxins in the organs and the cells, need to be flushed away in order to achieve a peaceful and healthy state.

THE FIVE REIKI PRINCIPLES

Dr Mikao Usui, who we know from the chapter on the history of Reiki healing is considered the originator of reiki, developed five reiki principles. It is believed that these were derived from the writings of the Emperor Meiji, the 122nd

Emperor of Japan who lived from 1852 to 1912.

The secret art of inviting happiness,

The miraculous medicine for all diseases.

At least for today:

Do not be angry,

Do not worry,

Be grateful,

Work with diligence,

Be kind to people.

Every morning and evening, join your hands in meditation and pray with your heart.

State in your mind and chant with your mouth.

For improvement of mind and body.

Usui Reiki Ryōhō.

The founder,

Mikao Usui.

It is believed that if you follow these simple steps you will have a more calming and balanced life.

AT LEAST FOR TODAY I WILL NOT BE ANGRY

This is a very simple thing to say, but in our busy and stressful lives practicing it is sometimes difficult. Our personal world is not always one of peace and harmony.

Negative feelings are said to create a serious blockage in our personal energy, which affects every aspect of our minds and souls. When we let go of anger, were are rewarded by inner peace and contentment.

AT LEAST FOR TODAY I WILL NOT WORRY

We all place worry on ourselves at some time or other. Some of us have become so good at living with worry that we no longer remember what life is like without it.

Filling our heads and hearts with worry only eats away at our body and soul. There will not be any peace or happiness in our lives if it is filled with worry.

When we let go of our worries, our minds are filled with a peace that brings inner healing and wellbeing.

AT LEAST FOR TODAY I WILL BE GRATEFUL

Feeling happy and well is always easier when we appreciate the things around us. By being grateful our spirit is raised and we feel good within our world.

If we are truly thankful from our hearts, the feeling will multiply the happiness in our lives.

Saying thank you, offering a smile to the people we pass or saying a kind word to our neighbors are small things. These small things will go a long way to making our hearts feel lighter and will help us to see the world in a more positive light.

A smile costs nothing, but gives so much in return.

AT LEAST FOR TODAY I WILL DO MY WORK DILIGENTLY

Most of us have to work to earn a living and it will truly help us if we can be happy doing the job we have. When we give our time honestly, we have peace within our working life.

If we make an honest attempt to treat our work and our employers with respect, only then will we feel accomplishment.

AT LEAST FOR TODAY I WILL BE KIND TO EVERY PERSON I MEET

Most of us feel that being kind is something we do all the time., but worry, stress and being upset can cause us to lose focus on how we behave towards the people around us.

When we are kind to our families, our co-workers, our elders and to strangers, we achieve a feeling of inner peace.

By being kind, we encourage the same in others. Kindness promotes a feeling of love that is much needed in the world.

REIKI SYMBOLS AND THEIR MEANINGS

Five symbols are used in the Usui reiki attunement process, during which the student's energy level is raised and the connection to universal spiritual energy is strengthened. The first four symbols are also used when reiki treatments are being performed.

These symbols do not hold any special powers in or of themselves, but were devised as teaching tools for reiki students to use when giving treatments and passing attunements. It is the intention that the practitioner has when using them that energizes the symbols.

THE POWER SYMBOL: CHO-KU-REI

Purposes: Manifestation, increased power, accelerated healing, catalyst for healing

Cho-Ku-Rei is used to increase the flow of reiki energy through the practitioner and increase the power of healing.

THE HARMONY SYMBOL: SEI-HEI-KI

Purposes: Cleansing, protection, mental and emotional healing

Sei-He-Ki is used for cleansing and purification, for protection, to clear negative energy, to release spirit attachments and in distant healing.

THE CONNECTION SYMBOL: HON-SHA-ZE-SHO-NEN

<u>Purposes</u>: Distant healing, healing karma, spiritual connection

Hon-Sha-Ze-Sho sends reiki through space and time and is used in all distant, past and future healing.

THE MASTER SYMBOL: DAI-KO-MYO

<u>Purposes</u>: Empowerment, soul healing, oneness

Dai-Ko-Myo is a powerful healing symbol and can also be used to cleanse and charge crystals and other objects.

THE COMPLETION SYMBOL: RAKU

<u>Purposes</u>: Kundalini healing, chakra alignment

Raku is only used during attunements. It is used to open up the new healer's energy channels and to separate the auras of the attuning master and the new healer.

BASIC REIKI HAND POSITIONS

The purpose of Reiki is to balance the body's energies in order to restore and promote good health and increase one's zest for life. In doing so, the Reiki hand positions are of great importance. There are nine positions. This article will briefly discuss what each of these positions are.

In the first position, the hands are placed upon the face. The palms of the hands go on either side of the face, forming a cup over the eyes, with the fingers touching the forehead. The touch needs to be gentle, applying no pressure.

In the second position, the hands rest on the top and crown of the head. The heel of each hand is placed on either side of the head close to the ears, with the fingertips resting on the crown.

For position three, the hands are placed behind the head. A cross is formed with the arms and one hand is placed above the nap of the neck and the other on the back of the head.

The fourth position concerns the collarbone and heart. The fingers and thumb of one hand are used to form a V and the neck is held in this V formation. The other hand rests between the heart and collarbone.

In the fifth position the chin and jaw are held. Hands are formed into a cup in which the chin rest. The hands are then extended to wrap over the jaw.

The ribs are included in the sixth position. One hand is placed on the upper part of the rib-cage, offering support to the elbow. The other hand rests on the abdomen with the fingertips touching the belly.

The seventh position concerns the pelvic region. The hands are placed on the pelvic bone with the fingertips touching the pelvic region.

The shoulders are the focus of the eighth position. With arms and elbows bent over the head, the hands rest first on the shoulder blades. While elbows remain bent, the hands are stretched down to touch the middle of the back.

The ninth position concerns the sacrum and lower back. The hands begin by resting gently on the lower back. Then they are lowered to rest on the sacral region.

Restoring energy flow and balance is the primary focus of reiki hand positions. It is not necessary to apply any pressure. A gentle touch is all that is needed to release any blocked energy.

REIKI BREATHING TECHNIQUES

The act of breathing is something many of us never think about as breathing just happens with no conscious effort on our part. In reiki it is believed that with the proper breathing technique we can aid in our journey to better health.

Breathing affects our whole body starting with the nervous system, the heart, the digestive system, muscles, sleep energy levels, concentration and memory to name just a few.

Most people breathe from the chest which is an uneconomical way to breathe as it only uses the top part of the chest and takes more muscle power. By only using the chest to breath we take more breaths and absorb less oxygen.

Take a deep breath slowly, release it and make an effort to judge the difference in how you feel. Many of us do this when we feel tired or stressed without thinking about it. This our bodies way of saying we are not looking after it.

The reiki technique of abdominal breathing teaches us to be kind to our bodies. This deep effective breathing begins with the breath starting in our abdomen and filling our whole body with life giving oxygen.

The practice begins with a clear mind and using the hands to aid in making the whole process become second nature. By placing our hands low on the abdomen we are able to judge how good our technique is.

Press gently and smoothly inward while expelling a breath for a count of six.

Hold for a count of two.

Release pressure smoothly while breathing in for a count of six.

Hold for a count of two.

These four steps of press hold and release are called a unit. After ten whole breathing units you should achieve a feeling of peace and calm. The most important part of this exercise is the press and release.

When you have mastered the physical aspects, visualize the release of negative energy when breathing out and drawing in positive energy when breathing in.

Breathing using the reiki technique is not hard but does take practice as we are used to breathing without conscious effort. It is worth persevering as it can be very beneficial to our health. If you find this difficult, a reiki practitioner can help with learning the correct technique.

Chapter 6: A View of the Usui Story

Much has been written about the life of Mikao Usui. The story that many of us were told in our First-degree classes has been challenged. Was Usui a doctor? Did he travel to the States? Was he Christian? The search for the historical Usui has been the subject of several books and the focus of much healthy debate. Now as interesting as these questions are, it is important not to become so involved with these details that vital aspects of the practice of Reiki are forgotten.

The beauty of Reiki is its simplicity; its simplicity in practice and its simplicity in teaching. Reiki teaching, up to the present, has been principally an oral tradition. The use of the word oral, although referring to the spoken word rather than the written, in the context of Reiki teaching refers to something rather more. Learning Reiki (if learning is in fact the right word) is about **being** and no amount of learning can bring this about. The quest for knowledge simply for its own sake is not enough. It just reinforces our reliance on the mind as a representation of who we are. This in turn maintains our sense of separateness, restricting us to its limits. All too often we judge a person (and ourselves) by what he has accumulated rather than by what he is.

Many teachers are shying away from telling the traditional Usui story through fear of ridicule in the light of the new details uncovered on Dr Usui.

In failing to explore this story an important part of the teaching of Reiki is missed. The Usui story, rather than being just a factual account of his life, is probably the second most important aspect of Reiki. In fact, if it were a choice of teaching the Usui story or the Reiki Principles I would rather teach the Usui story. Why? Because within the Usui story are all the principles and all the teachings of Reiki, in time-released form, (to use a current metaphor).

As we travel in the circle we refer to as our Reiki journey, we tell and retell this story. When we are ready, aspects of the story become clear. Rather than know the parts of the story we start to understand their teachings. It is the difference between knowledge and wisdom.

I said above that the story, in my opinion, is the second most important aspect of learning Reiki. What is the first then? ...doing it! I start my workshops with the old double question: you are walking along a path. On each side is thick mud. Cattle have used this path and added their contributions. As you walk, there in the biggest, muddiest and most gross area of the path you see a sparkle. You stop, bend down and to your amazement you find that it is a huge diamond. The two questions are; (1) do you bother to put your hand in and pick it up? And (2) is it any less valuable because it is covered in mud and the other stuff? So I tell the Reiki story and every now and then a little glimmer of light comes on helping me to stop trying to understand Reiki and just get on with it. I ask the folk I share my workshops with to meditate on the story or to re-read it and I try to share with them some of the jewels that are hidden within this story.

So let's share some of what I feel the Usui story tells us.

To start with, one of the Reiki principles that people have trouble with is the one that states: Honour your Teachers and Elders.

Usui was teaching when he was questioned by one of his students. This question was the catalyst that started him on his journey and in turn it gave us the practice we now call Reiki. The question arises therefore, who was the teacher? Which leads us on to: Who are our teachers? Everyone... Even the Bin Ladens and Sadam Hussein's of this world? Our reaction to the present situation can teach us a great deal about ourselves! Uhg!

As for our Elders? Well, I am learning the Djembe from a guy much younger than myself. He has been playing for years. In Djembe playing he is by far my elder. On another tack, looking at my 5-year-old grandson... He can certainly give me a lifetime or two. Who, therefore, are our elders?

His student's questions led Usui to realize that he did not have the answer. Admitting this and then doing something about it took courage.

Why courage? Well, most of us get to where we are through a mixture of luck and a great deal of hard work. The trouble is we work toward a goal conceived in ignorance. We create identities, gain status and credibility as we progress towards this goal. Putting into jeopardy all we have worked for takes courage. The fear of wasting all that time and energy blinds us to other possibilities. It is this fear that keeps us plodding along the same old path. And it is often this fear, the fear of losing what we have, our status and our hard earned positions, that keeps us form escaping the bonds of myths and illusions.

The three most precious words in the English language are….. "I don't know". By uttering these words you make the space for knowledge and then wisdom to come to you. Once you decide that you know or that you understand a thing, bang! the gate slams shut and rigidity sets in.

Usui set off to where he thought he would find the most up-to-date and complete information. The more he studied the more he realised he would not find what he needed. Current wisdom does not always mean the complete picture. Current thinking often throws the baby out with the bath water but it can help us to formulate the questions needed. It is the questions rather than the answers that are important. Answers are current and static. Time changes many things. Questions on the other hand generate movement.

Returning to his native land he looked elsewhere, freeing himself of single-track thinking and at last he found what he was looking for.

But knowledge alone is not enough. How many times do we find ourselves suddenly understanding something that we have known for ages? It is as if we shift into another gear and **ping** on goes the light, often taking us completely by surprise.

Really understanding needs something more than just facts.

Living in his culture and being of his time, up he went onto the mountain determined to solve the problem, to sit there until all became clear. Twenty-one days was the time set. As each day passed... nothing. No matter how well he sat, no matter how hard he tried, no matter how much he meditated nothing came to him. The twenty-one days passed. Still nothing! All that hard work, all that studying, all that sitting and still nothing. He threw away the last stone and with it his attachment to finding the answer and at the very moment of surrender he saw a light.

By releasing the thought of being in control of the learning process he made room for true understanding to shine through. Still he hesitated, fear still holding him, fear of the unknown, of letting go, of trusting in his true self. Worrying about all of this would have made him duck or avoid the approaching ball of light. (Now, in the Principles we teach, it says "Just for today I will not worry". I think today is too long a time. All that is needed is to replace today with **Now**. Now is where we are meant to be. Now keeps us in the only time that has any relevance. It also leads to the next Now.) But he did not move, he let go of his final attachment, even that of his own life.

Wham! The light struck him full on. Bubbles containing the symbols flooded his brain; the physical manifestation of Reiki. After a time his return to a more physical reality revealed that he understood what he had known before. This **instant** enlightenment had taken years to achieve. All we have to do is accept our place in Reiki to rid ourselves of the illusions we have worked on for so long. The moment of realisation might be instantaneous but getting there can take time. Our practise in Reiki (or rather The Usui System of Natural Healing, for we are Reiki rather than practising it) helps loosen the bonds that hold these illusions tight until suddenly they just fall away and we find ourselves as we always have been... perfect.

We have been given a gift so precious that most of us take it for granted. In fact many of us spend our time trying to avoid it, to escape it. It is the gift of a physical body and a physical world. These are the tools we have to work with and which we should make the most of. It is great to escape for a while to live up our mountain. But Usui's story tells us to come back down and get back in the place where we are meant to be even if it means banging your toe, like Usui. Without the pain he would not have known what he could do.

This brings us neatly to the so-called Reiki miracles. When I first heard of them I was, to say the least, rather underwhelmed. They were small and hardly worth mentioning. I wanted real miracles. Sea-parting, raising-the-dead type miracles. Toe stubbing, toothache and eating food, to my mind, were not very impressive.

And that is one of the problems of the time in which we live. We have been so conditioned to look for the extravaganzas that our eyes are fixed on the horizon looking for the big miracle, all celestial choirs and Wurlitzers. We miss the thousands of miracles that happen all around us every day. We need to stop and look, really look. Which brings us right back to Reiki.

Usui found that he could help people on the physical level, to heal the beggars of their pains. Helping them fit into society, to be a useful part of that society and so live happy and productive lives. He worked tirelessly. Giving of himself, never asking reward until one day he was forced to face the fact that people were returning to the beggar community. He fell down distraught. Not angry with those who were returning, despite all he had done. Distraught that he had failed to see the full picture. We cannot decide what path a person should take or what their needs are. They must do this for themselves. Our definition of healing is ours alone, with all the limitations it carries with it. It is not enough to heal just the physical. We are, by far, much more. The emotional, the mental and the spiritual, all must come into balance. The desire to change needs to be on all these levels for real healing to take place. But more important is the realisation that there are no different levels, no one to heal and no healing needed.

Unafraid, Usui learned from this experience and off he went again, borrowing and revising a set of guidelines, setting himself up for ridicule by wandering around with his lamp. Promoting himself in the same way in order to give people a chance to share in his understanding. His love for all beings shining through the darkness.

In the darkest cave, deep down where no sun shines, a single candle will push back the darkness. Two candles will do a better job. A thousand will fill the space with light. The darkness can never put out even one of those candles. The only thing that can return the darkness is letting the candles go out. Fear, hate and ignorance are the best ways of snuffing out those candles.

All that is written here is "my mud". Deep down in it, I hope, is at least the glimmer of that precious diamond.

Is the Usui Story true? If we continue to tell it, the answer is yes. Let us tell it with love and with fun. See Usui rushing down the mountain, robes flowing, stubbing his toe, hopping around cursing, until suddenly, in wonder the pain stops. Feel his despair as he throws away that last stone. Go on to tell of Hayashi and Takata, for within their stories are also lessons if only we look into our hearts and find them.

Well, having got that out of the way, on we go…….

Chapter 7: What Being a Reiki Teacher / Attuner Involves

After being with Reiki for a while many feel the urge to 'TEACH' it to others. In our humble experience the only way for Reiki to be passed on is to LIVE it as deeply and wholly as is humanly possible.

These ideals seem valid at this time:

Honesty
Openness
Purity
Energy

These are the four elements most needed for positive healing, from both the channelled and the person seeking help. Try using them and miracles will happen. Allow Reiki to transform your life and the lives of many you attune.

Payment / Money

What to charge for our services is a concern to many. Ask yourself what are **your** needs and motives.

o   Is your intention to spread Reiki as far as possible whatever the cost to yourself and family?

o   Do you expect to make a fortune from your time?

o   Are you content to take a middle path?

Our advice is to do whatever feels right for **you.** There are always plenty ready to advise you. Listen if you wish but in the end be confident enough to make your own decisions. Always remember to change your mind as you progress onward. What is your truth today may very well be outdated tomorrow. Endeavour to stay balanced throughout.

It is a great commitment to become a full Reiki Teacher. There will be many challenges and adversities to overcome as your own growth develops alongside those you attune. As we welcome your dedication as a teacher /attuner/master in the Usui Reiki tradition, we realise the humility of the nature and quality of this kind of work. We trust you will, as we try to do, leave "self" behind when you enter into the attunement space. Dr Usui put himself under immense pressure in an endeavour to gain the truth of healing. He realised eventually it is only when **we** step back and allow Universal Love to flow through unimpeded that the miracles start to happen. Let us honour his memory by doing the same.

Practical Considerations and Useful Tips

Make sure you have an elementary knowledge of anatomy. Let people know what part of the body they are touching and how the physical level treatment affects them. Give people an embodied, "breathed into" sense of the energy pathways in the body. Be confident in doing this.

Introduce maps of the body - chakras, meridians, auras, etc., if you are familiar with them [see previous books]. This can be done as you teach the hand positions. Always show people how to give a treatment and give them plenty of time to practise.

Encourage participants to drink lots of water during the days of the workshop and several days after. This will assist physical well-being.

Introduce the issue of "taking the next step towards being the healer" as a topic for reflection and thought. Hold a quiet space for this to happen in.

Your own meditation techniques can be introduced. Meditations that call in the Reiki masters and other helpers can assist too.

Have handbooks or your own written material available as examples. Combine this with some storytelling and lots of hands-on practice creating a receptive climate for the attunements. Suggest that people spend a quiet evening after the attunements. Ask them to stay in the energy and to pay attention to their dreams and meditations.

Ask participants to practice Reiki daily, note their experiences and write to you after 21 days to record something of their experiences. This replicates Dr Usui's meditation, and further links people with the tradition. It is also nourishing for us to appreciate our contribution.

As you attune people to Reiki be mindful of their state of self worth. They need anchors to believe they are receiving the gift. The attunements themselves and the circle we create in setting the stage for our classes provide that anchor.

Reiki is quite fashionable at this time. Do make sure folk fully understand their commitment. Get them to verbalise their readiness to take the step into Reiki. Emphasise to the receiver it is their choice, not yours, to be attuned.

Attunements can do no harm but may start off a process some are not consciously ready to deal with. Attunements can be quite physically tiring to give. Take care of yourselves as well as those coming to you. Allow the process to develop as you do too.

Maybe start with small numbers allowing the numbers to grow as your confidence and stamina does. [I once slept through lunchtime when I had over-stretched myself.] Have an assistant, trainee or co-teacher to take on some of the workload and to laugh at your jokes!!

Try to avoid adding long journeys to the class time. Travel the previous day if necessary.

Do also keep to the agenda of simply Reiki. It gets very complicated if Reiki attunements are combined or tacked on to other activities. Ensure that the group understands this. Having Reiki attunements combined with reflexology during the lunch break can take the individual into overload and detract from the focus of Reiki. Be aware of the few who hijack the class to promote themselves, not healing.

With taking on the role of teaching Reiki to others we enter into another stage of our own personal journey. There have been many great masters and teachers before us. It is part of our duty in honouring Reiki to maintain high standards. Trying to live daily by these principals in all that we do allows us to become more effective channels of Universal life force. In turn we can pass this state onto other beings.

Placing the chairs so there is room to comfortably walk all around each individually is desirable. However one should always be adaptable. If it feels right to attune each one individually then do so. We have attuned sick people in bed with good outcome!

Setting the group energy, the physical scene, with music or silence, incense, lights etc. is all a matter of choice. Let your inner knowing lead you in this.

We all get ideas of Healing the World. Why not heal ourselves as thoroughly as we can and let the world follow our example and benefit?

Reiki connects us up with a true potential of human <u>being</u>. We thank all our sources, Reiki Masters, Dr Usui, Dr Hayashi, Mrs Takata, Martha, Sandi and most of all Yamura. She encouraged us to simply be ourselves. We thank you all who come to us for healing.

A blessing on our circle ever increasing.

Chapter 8: What are the Five Precepts?

GOKAI/REIKI PRECEPTS: THE RULES OF CONDUCT

For Today Only:
- Do Not Anger
- Do Not Worry
- Be Humble
- Be Honest In Your Work
- Be Compassionate To Yourself And Others

~ Translated by Chris Marsh

WHAT ARE PRECEPTS?

A precept is a code of practice. Usui provided these principles to deepen the practice of self-healing. They were given to provide a complete foundation within the system of Reiki, becoming a guide for living and healing. Should one focus daily on these words, the spiritual transformation and awareness would indeed be quickly experienced. The precepts are a simple and effective tool to change your self-image by rejecting any untruths you have claimed as your reality.

According to **The Japanese Art of Reiki,** by Bronwen and Frans Stiene, Usui formed a creed as an introduction to The Five Precepts :

The precepts are a simple and effective tool to change your selfimage by rejecting any untruths you have claimed as your reality.

"The secret of inviting happiness through many blessings, the spiritual medicine for all illness."

The explanation continues: "Do gassho every morning and evening, keep in your mind and recite." **The system's goal is then acknowledged:** "Improve your mind and body."

Mind and body are part of our human selves. These are considered to be the two diamonds. As they become balanced, a third diamond is created to represent the spirit. You become like a sparkling, multi-faceted diamond, shining and revealing your creative infinite TRUE self.

The closing of the creed, **Usui Reiki Ryoho**, emphasizes the name of the healing method, translated literally as "Usui Spiritual Healing Method."

ORIGIN OF THE FIVE PRECEPTS

Usui based The Five Precepts from Japanese Buddhism, specifically The Eight-Fold Path. It instills in a practitioner the following: right views, right thinking, right speech, right action, right way of life, right endeavor, right mindfulness and right meditation.

Dr. Usui molded these codes into a non-religious form. When he began teaching these around 1915, students were encouraged to write the precepts to internalize the meanings.

The reign of the Shinto Meiji Emperor (1852-1912) also had an influence on Dr. Usui. The emperor impressed upon his people "Five Principles" to improve the quality of their lives. Dr. Usui recognized their importance to help remove suffering and disease.

As the precepts become second nature, their influence is absorbed

 into all of your actions.

BENEFITS OF THE FIVE PRECEPTS

When practicing the precepts, you are inadvertently reminded of the presence of "now" time. You begin to change your mind set. An "attitude adjustment" takes place and your situations begin to change accordingly. You become what you think.

As the precepts become second nature, their influence is absorbed into all of your actions. How can you become enmeshed in past issues and blame when you refocus your attention to the present moment? It is healthier and wise to let those memories and emotions serve as a lesson. Only then can you catapult yourself into new worthwhile experiences. When visions of lack and challenges begin to drain and weigh you down, immediately recite **The Five Precepts**. It allows you to tap into your divine potential and to release your inner power. As a whole, **The Five Precepts** deepen your process of healing and self discovery.

PRACTICING THE FIVE PRECEPTS

A regular minimal practice with **The Five Precepts** is reciting them aloud, morning and evening, in gassho (prayer pose). You may either stand or sit in seiza (rock pose). Feel the emotions and higher energetic vibrations behind the words. Enjoy the strength of your voice and allow the power within you, to join with the power of your spoken word. Multiple repetitions throughout the day reinforce their energy. A deeper connection is formed, which naturally pulls you away from distress and angst. You are forming a relationship with these new codes to assist you in living your life to its fullest. Additionally, reciting them aloud strengthens your energy field, or aura. This is especially helpful before beginning a healing.

After a few days of morning and evening contemplation, begin writing the precepts by hand. Your arms are the extension of your heart. Writing allows you to imprint them more deeply into your subconscious. A familiarity begins to develop. When you write them and place in visible areas, your mind is prevented from straying into the negative zone. You are exposing yourself to the development of new possibilities.

VISUALIZING THE FIVE PRECEPTS

Take a moment after each precept to envision their impact on your life. See yourself moving through the day with ease, being fully available to the moment. Your thoughts and words are "things" which create your reality. Choose wisely by being guided by **The Five Precepts**. Let the following quote further your understanding on the importance of holding clear meaningful images:

"The vision that you glorify in your mind, The Ideal that you enthrone in your heart: This you will build your life by, This you will become."
~ James Allen, As A Man Thinketh
THE SIGNIFICANCE OF "JUST FOR TODAY"
I understand the past and its memories are behind me.
I openly accept the gifts and relevant messages that each precept brings.

Just for today , I am centered in the present moment that holds immense possibilities for me. I attract certain conditions based on the quality of my thoughts. I am encouraging myself to expect more from life.

I keep a clear perspective of who I am. I do not settle on things just the way they appear to be. I enthusiastically visualize them as they can be. I hold successful images in my mind. My life begins to transform to one of balance and abundance.

I am changing my consciousness and expanding my awareness. I am synchronized with the flow of the universe. I am a spiritual warrior in charge of my life.

Walt Whitman's poem succinctly expresses this:
Oh, while I live, to be the ruler of life, not a slave,

to meet life as a powerful conqueror,
And nothing exterior to me shall ever take command of me.

I. Just for today, I do not anger

Can I be peaceful and calm today?

I allow myself to breathe in the fullness of life. I am centered in the glory of who I am. I am an "instrument of peace," possessing the peace that passeth all understanding. I am poised in this peace.

Anger is an out-of-control emotion. Anger is a signal that I am off-balance. I find ways to safely clear myself of this and not suppress the emotion. For a moment, I place my attention on the anger and observe it. I feel it without judgment. In doing so, I am being non-resistant and find ways to safely clear it. I am willing to release and let go. I re-center into my truth. I understand that whatever I resist persists. I continually practice the art of relaxing, surrendering and releasing. I am now in charge!

II. Just for today, I do not worry

What if worry really took flight from my world today and vanished? If so, I believe that desirable conditions can be created by me. I am now aware that worry brings on fear and depletes my good. I begin to reverse this process and see myself being calm and centered with a positive vision of my day.

Just for today, I have faith. Any fears are cleared at the moment of recognition. I conserve my inner Ki, optimum health and wellness **just for today**. There is a divine flow that is always present. When I believe in my visions, I am connected to Source energy. I sometimes "act as if" to stay in tune with this creative flow. As I recite this precept, I truly know I am a spiritual being, having my place in an abundant Universe. I am a unique child in this creative process. I am ME.

I understand that whatever I resist persists. I continually practice the art of relaxing, surrendering and releasing. I am now in charge!
I am a blessing to the world. I move from one joyous situation to the next.

III. Just for today, I am grateful

"A grateful mind is a great mind which eventually attracts to itself great things."
~ Plato

My gratefulness is like an inner lighthouse shining radiance onto my paths **just for today**. When my heart is filled with gratitude, I further open the way to synchronicities. I become an attractive force field that draws to itself great things.

I live each day with a grateful heart, one day at a time and I am filled with greatness. As I feel grateful, I become charming to my environment. I become "irresistibly divine" to my highest good. I am releasing an energy that pulls opportunities to me. I am like a magnet that attracts plenty of good back to me. In this state of constant thanksgiving, I am able to find good in all my situations. There is something I can be thankful for in any challenge and lesson.

Just for today, I am a blessing to the world. I move from one joyous situation to the next.

IV. Just for today, I work honestly

"No matter what your work, let it be your own.
No matter what your occupation, let what you are doing be organic. Let it be in your bones. In this way you will open the door

by which the affluence of heaven and earth
shall stream into you."
~ Ralph Waldo Emerson "Let the beauty of what you love, be what you do."
~ Rumi

My work is more than "just a living." It is an opportunity to make a life for myself. My life is a growth process. I do my very best to serve, to give of my unique talents and gifts. What I "feel in my bones," as indicated by Ralph Waldo Emerson, is joy, aliveness, awareness, and meaningful service. I discipline myself everyday to put more Ki into each phase of my work. This contributes to my growth and knowing myself, my truth. Thus, I know the Universe is guiding me in my affairs so I may sing my very own heart's song.

V. Just for today, I am kind and compassionate

"If you want others to be happy, practice compassion. If you want to be happy, practice compassion."
Tenzin Gyatso (14th Dalai Lama)

I am part of the Universal Mind. I forgive those I perceive to have "wronged" me. This clears my own field of consciousness. I am able to accept people and things as they are. I send forth love and bless the people in my life and all circumstances. The act of blessing changes me and my outlook. It increases the flow of good into my life.

This leads to acceptance of what is and who is in my life. It allows me to release any judgments of myself and others, just for today.

The act of blessing changes me and my outlook. It increases the flow of good into

my life.

Chapter 9: Fifteen Reasons to Apply Reiki to Your Own Life

Reiki aids in the healing of any unpleasant issue in your life, be it a mental or physical problem. Reiki clients have enjoyed astonishing results, and listed below are some benefits that you could also take advantage of:

Makes complete relaxation of the body possible, which helps release tension in the body.

Accelerates your body's automatic healing system.

Sleep patterns improve.

Blood pressure decreases, relieving other health problems.

Helps acute, as well as chronic health problems, from mild injuries to asthma to migraines, and assists in ridding addictions.

Relieves pains.

Blockages of energy are removed, which adjusts the flow of energy in the endocrine system, transferring the body into an instrument of harmony.

Cleans the body of its toxins.

Helps with the recovery from chemical therapies after surgery and medical prescriptions, diminishing the side effects from these drugs.

Boosts immune system.

Slows down aging, and increases vigour.

Increases vibrational rate in the body.

Grows spirituality and purifies the emotions.

Reinforces alternative medicine means such as crystals and acupuncture, and intensifies health care received from modern health care practitioners.

Develops better relationships, making time spent with loved ones more productive and enjoyable.

Reiki Principles

Five Spiritual Principles

Reiki is a tool for gaining spiritual enlightenment. Reiki can heal physically, mentally, emotionally and spiritually. Those who are already familiar with Reiki energy healing concepts are probably aware of the five Spiritual Principles as well. These are to be practiced in your daily life during your thoughts, deeds and words instead of them simply being recited and memorised. Living these five principles will give your life new meaning, and complete satisfaction and happiness in life. The five principles are listed below:

1. Anger Release

"Just for today, I will not be angry."

Anger at yourself or anyone else leads to energy blockages. Anger is an enemy that emanates from inside us. Reiki helps remove the blockages created from anger, but cannot prevent future blockages from the anger that later flares up. It is wise to let all anger free from our minds so as not to let the energy blockages return.

2. Worry Release

"Just for today, I will not worry."

Worry comes from negative thoughts about future events. Worrying may not always be negative, but chronic worrying creates tension and can poison your body, mind and soul. Ridding the mind of worry through Reiki requires the positive energy flow to be distributed throughout the body. Freeing the mind of worry enables healing to enter the body.

3. Gratitude

"Just for today, I will be grateful."

Being genuinely grateful is great for healing. Your intentions are imperative in this exercise. Simply being grateful, forgiving others, and taking nothing for granted increases your quality of life, and does the same for those around you. This lets joy fill your spirit.

4. Honesty

"Just for today, I will do my work honestly."

Work honestly, and give yourself and your family the support you both need. This means doing work that does not intend to harm others. Living an honorable life, and working diligently, so it brings happiness into your life.

5. Kindness

"Just for today, I will be kind to every living thing."

Honour your family, teachers, parents, elders, friends and every living being around you. Being a kind person enables love to enter the soul.

Searching for the Reiki Teacher

Qualities to Look For

Treatment procedures

Credentials

Number of clients treated

Where they were trained in Reiki, and by whom

Positive feedback from past clients

Where to Search

Searching in the yellow pages of your phone book will not likely help you find a Reiki teacher. Many do not advertise their ministry, and instead, typically work from hospitals, clinics, spas or their own homes. Many do not participate in house calls or travel anywhere for treatment purposes. Bulletin boards at natural health stores, yoga classes and colleges are sometimes a good source for finding Reiki practitioners. They typically rely on word of mouth to gain business. Be sure to ask many questions to ensure that you are getting the Reiki style you prefer, as there are many different styles used by different practitioners.

Research

When conducting research via the internet, information can be contradicting at times. This is because there are many different divisions in Reiki, which results in many different philosophies and techniques used in the art. Though the contradictory information is sometimes confusing, the various viewpoints can be helpful in deciding which form of Reiki is most suitable to you. The internet can also help you find the nearest group of Reiki enthusiasts that you could join.

Chapter 10: Taoist System Of The Five Phases Of The Chi Cycle

The Chinese concept of bioenergy is Chi. Chi is the thread of union that crosses everything in the Universe but does not have a definite form. Chi flows and is constantly transformed, manifests itself in innumerable aspects and is the origin of all life and manifestation. Chi is a general concept. The different manifestations of Chi receive specific names to indicate the qualities that it adopts and the functions that it fulfills in each moment. We can understand this better if we study Taoist cosmogony (formation of the universe) a bit.

Chi-Wu

Chi-Wu would be the previous universe in which there is nothing differentiated. There is no way or distinguish any being.

Only chi. It is the primal emptiness. For beings to appear and take shape, differentiation is necessary. The understanding of this state of Chi escapes our capacity. We can compare it with an empty space with the potential to create everything that exists in the Universe.

Yin and Yang

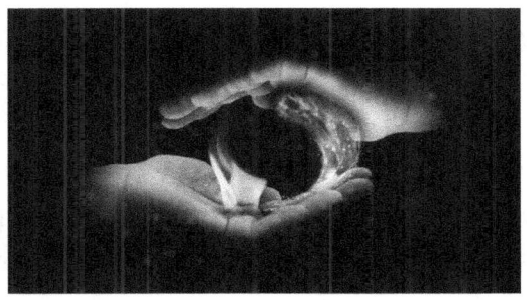

For the forms that make up the Universe to exist, there must be something that breaks the conformity of Chi-Wu. The differentiation that makes one manifestation different from the other must appear. Chi has to manifest itself in a differentiated way: on the one hand the apparent and on the other the hidden, on the one hand, the tangible and on the other, the intangible. It is the manifestation of duality. This dual differentiation of the manifestations of the Universe is represented by Yin and Yang.

Movement and change are inherent in the concept of Yin and Yang. Yin and Yang are the result of the first movement of the Universe and only exist when there is movement. Yang grows to the point where it begins to become Yin and this, in turn, will follow the same process to return to Yang. If Chi finds the perfect balance on his way between the Yin and Yang, then the movement would stop and Chi would return to the original void, Chi-Wu, as there was no differentiation. Nature reproduces in its cycles this cycle of Chi:

The seasons of the year, the traffic between day and night, the life and death cycles of living beings and everything in the universe is subjected to this dance.

Yin and Yang are the two pillars of all manifestation: the two basic aspects under which Chi can manifest itself, differentiating itself and acting by contrast and complementarity: thus we will have what "is" versus what "is not," belonging to the spirit against what belongs to the physical world, the hot versus the cold, the soft versus the hard, the expansive versus the contractive, the destructive versus the constructive, etc. These two forms of manifestation are relative and interdependent and are never absolute. In a given being we will always find the Yin and Yang interacting to endow that being with its own characteristics.

Yin is

the solid

the heavy

the cold

the motionless

the dense

the matter

the physical

Yang is

the hollow

the light

the hot

the dynamic

the subtle

the energy

the spiritual

The Three Pure Forces

After differentiation, Yin and Yang will manifest in different degrees through different forms of existence. Chi will manifest in its maximum Yin degree in solid, cold and stable bodies. On the other hand, the most Yang manifestations of Chi will be found in the intangible, in the most subtle and imperceptible energies. On the one hand, we have the most solid and stable bodies, which tend to coldness and inertia. On the other hand, we have pure energy, which in many cases is so subtle that it does not have an apparent influence on solid matter.

Between one extreme and another, we find an infinity of forms of manifestation of energy and matter with different degrees of structuring. Through these intermediate scales the more subtle manifestations of Chi affect those that are somewhat denser and these in turn to the following until more physical energies are able to directly affect matter (Yang governs the Yin) but it is necessary a large amount of energy affect a solid mass, so that solid bodies (Yin) accumulate large amounts of energy (Yang) before being affected by it (Yin retains Yang).

The Taoists divided the scale from Chi plus Yin to most Yang into three large sections. These are the Three Pure Forces that feed and give life to the rest of the manifestations, the three main manifestations of Chi.

This representation of the universe is a conception that takes man as the center. In reality we can summarize the idea of the three pure forces so that the Celestial Chi would be the one who exerts his influence on us from the sky, the Cosmic

Chi would be the one that constitutes the game of life in the terrestrial biosphere, and the Telluric Chi they would be the influences of the planet itself on us and the biosphere.

Chi Celeste is the most spiritual manifestation of Chi in the Universe. It is the Chi that remains in a more ethereal state, almost without evolving into the matter. This Chi affects increasingly dense manifestations until it affects the physical plane. The stars are magnificent entrance doors of the Chi Celeste in the physical plane. In the stars, large quantities of matter diluted in large quantities of the energy of different densities are found. In them, the impact of the Celestial Chi on the matter could be almost immediate.

Cosmic Chi is the physical manifestations of the Celestial Chi that have not adopted a material entity. It is the Chi that has a greater capacity for metamorphosis. It is

Chi in the middle of the path of evolution between spirit and matter, in one way or another. The physical forces, the different sources of energy and influences that we receive from the bodies of our environment make up the Cosmic Chi. This is the type of Chi that maintains the game of life as we know it and, on whose balance, our physical-emotional health depends.

Telluric Chi is the Chi manifested on our planet. The Chi immobilized almost completely in material form and whose almost exclusive source for the Human Being is the Earth. It is the matter of it, but also its radiation and denser energies. For human beings, the most absolute Yin force by which it is influenced is our dear Planet Earth. Planet Earth gives us the Yin, the physical manifestation.

The interaction of the Three Pure Forces makes life appear, which is the result of the influence of the Celestial Chi (spirit) on the Telluric Chi (matter) generating the Cosmic Chi (vital energy). The Three Pure Forces are a consequence of the polarization of Chi (Yin and Yang).

Chapter 11: The Solar Plexus Chakra

The Solar Plexus Chakra is responsible for mental power. It governs your ability to comprehend and learn. It governs will power as well as the ego. It emits confidence and optimism. If you wish to align your Solar Plexus Chakra you must be able to concentrate and focus. You must examine your life to find out if you lack confidence and rely on what other people think of you to provide self worth. Furthermore, you must determine if you are having a hard time deciding because you thoughts are clouded. It is also possible that you may have a lot of responsibilities because you believe you know best. You should determine if you are a perfectionist and are the type of person that prefers to do everything yourself. Lastly, you must know if you are afraid of being alone.

You can boost this chakra center and take in yellow energy by engaging in mind puzzles, informative books, and classes. You can develop your photographic memory and enroll in detoxification programs. Yellow is the color of the Solar Plexus Chakra so eating and drinking yellow colored foods is crucial. Aromatherapy oils like bergamot, grapefruit, lemon, and rosemary are good for this chakra center. Horn and reed instruments as well as chimes are music which stimulates the Solar Plexus Chakra. Gemstones like Topaz, Amber and Citrine as well as gold must be carried or worn. Lastly, arts, color baths, decors, and clothing must also be in yellow.

The Solar Plexus Chakra resides in the stomach area, just above the navel. Its Sanskrit name is Manipura. This chakra is responsible for the sense of personal power. It balances ego power, self-confidence, and intellect. It helps in the ability to develop a sense of humor and self control. If there is an imbalance in the Solar Plexus Chakra, the you may have poor memory, colitis, parasites, toxicity, nervousness, constipation, hypoglycemia, diabetes, ulcers, and digestive problems. This chakra is connected to large parts of the body like the muscular system, the solar plexus, the skin, the large intestine, the liver, the stomach, and other glands and organs near the solar plexus. Furthermore, the eyes and the face are part of this chakra because the face is what shows to the world. The pancreas is the connected endocrine gland.

In terms of consciousness, the Solar Plexus chakra is associated with perceptions of ease of being, freedom, control, and power. The mental sphere and activity are also part of this chakra. In most cases, the ego or the personality is the closest association of this chakra to the level of being. Because of the relationship with the sun or with fire, this chakra also represents the relationships of the human being with the other parts of his consciousness. As such, if you have sensitivities with the sun, you also are sensitive about freedom, control, or power.

Since the sense of sight is associated with the Solar Plexus Chakra, a person with impaired vision is said to be experiencing tensions at this chakra. You could also have issues about freedom, control, and power. If you nearsighted, you also may be tensed around the solar plexus. You may feel insecure or experience fear. On the other hand, a farsighted individual has problems with the throat chakra and may feel guilt or anger. A person who has astigmatism is said to be confused.

The pancreas is the associated endocrine gland with this chakra center. A person who has diabetes is said to be keeping sweetness from themselves. If someone wants to get close to this person, they may feel threatened. In general, diabetes is related to the suppression of anger.

The Solar Plexus Chakra emits confidence. If it is open, you will feel dignified and in control. If it's under-active, you may feel indecisive and passive. Frequently, you may feel as if you aren't rewarded which makes you feel apprehensive. If the chakra is overactive, you could become aggressive and imperious.

To open the Solar Plexus Chakra, you must feel relaxed while sitting on your knees with your back straight. Your hands must be put before your stomach, just below the solar plexus. The fingers must point away from you and must join at the top. The thumbs must be crossed with the fingers straightened. Next, you must concentrate on the meaning of the Solar Plexus Chakra then chants "RAM" clearly yet silently. You must be more relaxed while still thinking about the chakra and its meaning to your life. You must maintain the position until you feel completely relaxed.

Chapter 12: CHAKRAS – The Energy Centres

6.1. Activate the Seven Energy Centres

Man should activate all the seven energy centres if he has to head himself. (Refer to the chart of energy centres in Appendix)

6.1.1. Crown or Turiya

Starting from the head, the first chakra is sahasraara. Position of the pineal gland, this is the holistic position of the thousand petalled lotus. The pineal gland secretes the melatonin hormone.

6.1.2. Temple

Ajna chakra – abode of Sadashiva. Position of the pituitary gland which secretes 10 hormones. Students desirous to study well should activate these two glands to perfection.

6.1.3. Neck

Visuddha is the chakra. This is where the thyroid and parathyroid glands are situated.

6.1.4. Chest

The heart's energy centre is Anahata. Thymus gland is situated here.

6.1.5. Belly Button

Above this on the left side, lies the Manipura chakra. This gland here secretes insulin, which successfully combats sugar in blood. Being the birthplace of anger, it is referred to as the Balipeeda holistically. This is the place where the hands are placed at the time of veneration.

6.1.6. Reproductive Organs

The chakra is called svadhishtaana and the glands, testes and ovary are present here.

in men and women, respectively. **6.1.7. Mooladhara**

At the fag end of the spine resides the holistic serpent shaped power of Kundalini. The chakra is called Mooladhara. The adrenal gland is based here.

If a man activates these seven energy centres, he can lead a life of health and prosperity. And this activation becomes possible with the adoption of cosmic energy.

Our ancestors have taken acute care and acumen in designing our lives in a practical way in consonance with nature. Indian tradition has rich values and boasts of a scientific explanation for each ritual which is aimed to create a positive change in a human. And, we humans at large adopt and practise certain rituals blindly without understanding the reality behind them. For instance, Indians advocate certain methods and exercises to keep good health and spirits.

6.2. The Energy Centres, Their Colours in Cosmic Energy Therapy

6.2.1. Sahasraara – Turiya – Crown – Violet

House of the thousand petalled lotus, this is the place of the pineal gland that secretes melatonin. The colour attributed to this chakra is violet or white.

6.2.2. Ajna – Pituitary Gland – Temple – Indigo or Dark Blue

Termed as a master gland, this gland secretes 10 hormones. For the body and brain to function properly, these hormones should function accurately. The food goes to the brain through the blood. A proper implementation of cosmic energy makes your face glow with divine resplendence, unless you have not practiced it properly. If the face is sans glow, it should be understood that blood flow to the brain is not proper.

A master teaching cosmic energy radiates the divinity of a Buddha. An increased blood flow radiates the face with resplendence and, in my personal experience; I have seen many such people getting radiated after cosmic energy therapy and initiation.

Take, for instance, the energy centre of ajna, the temple. If a person (usually ajna chakra is situated in the front of head and at the back of it) has the ajna opened in the front and closed in the back, he cannot be a practical man. He may be proficient with many concepts, but will not implement anything completely. The colour of this chakra is dark blue.

6.2.3. Visuddhi – Thyroid – Throat – Blue

The blue colour has the power to pacify a wavering mind. A mere glance of the sky and the blue sea tranquillizes one's mind. Further, blue dresses soothe oneself.

Placing a hand on the throat and imagining blue colour make us experience the increased flow of cosmic energy. The thyroid g and is responsible for keeping a good physique. Lack of thyroid gland's potency makes a man look obese.

Some may be lean, the reason being the excessive working of the thyroid gland. Based on the thyroid gland's performance, we can ascertain the efficiency, performance and ability of an employee in an office.

6.2.4. Heart - Green

Green is the colour attributed to the heart's energy centre. Some parents may have seeded unnecessary and baseless fears about the existence of evil spirits and demons in their child's mind. As the child grows up, he/she may feel insecure when alone or amidst strangers. When people approach me to protect them from evil spirits, I elucidate on the reality and treat them for their baseless fears.

Only a disturbed mind can conceive unfounded fears in demons, ogresses and evil spirits. Hence, tranquillity of mind is essential. For this, placing of green or rose coloured stones on the chest radiates to dispel the baseless fears and instils confidence.

I travel the length and breadth of India by train. When I feel restless, I place my hands on my chest and infuse cosmic energy. This puts me to sleep, that too a sound one. Only in the morning do I wake up, refreshed, from having slept well.

The most common disease today is insomnia. To soothe the heart's energy centre and manipura, place your hands on them and activate them.

6.2.5. Belly – Yellow

The color of yellow is attributed to the manipura chakra. Around 10 crore people are affected by sugar around the world. Classified into two, that is, blood sugar caused by insulin and blood sugar not related to insulin, this disease can be effectively curtailed by channelising cosmic energy to the manipura chakra.

6.2.6. Mooladhara - Red

When the Mooladhara is weak, a red stone is used to cure it. Even keeping a red stone in the hands cures the malfunctioning of the Mooladhara. 90% of the people complain of pain in the spine and this can be controlled by strengthening of the Mooladhara with cosmic energy.

6.2.7. Orange – Svadhishthana

The svadhishthana chakra has the colour of orange as its attribute.

A constant practice of infusing cosmic energy on the seven energy centres keeps them in good shape and protects the body from diseases. These centres of energy are the storehouse of worldly principles.

As Albert Einstein observed: "Even scientists are spiritualists. Only when they are spiritualists, could they invent admirable inventions."

It is this statement that has become the underlying factor for today's worldly existence. No counter-statement and protests can be made, for this is the ultimate truth.

Science and spiritualism are one and the same. **6.3. The Deities in the Chakras**

The underlying crux of Indian scriptures is the six centres of energy in Mooladhara, svadhishthana, manipura, anahata, visuddhi and ajna. These six centres of energy have six presiding deities in each one of them.

6.3.1. Kandar Anubhuthi

One should cross all the six centres of energy to reach the pinnacle. Lord Muruga, the six-faced Supreme Being, is the presiding deity of these six energy centres.

Realisation of God is attained when these six energy centres are in good shape. Each energy centre has a presiding deity for it. Lord Ganapathi is the presiding deity for the first energy centre (chakra) of Mooladhara, Lord Brahma for Svathishtaanaa, Lord Vishnu for Manipoorakaa, Lord Rudra for Anagathaa, Lord Maheswara for Visucdhi and Lord

Sadasiva for the penultimate chakra of Ajna.

The Seventh chakra is Sahasrara which is the centre of enfoldment of this supreme realisation.

6.4. Seven Everywhere

The Cosmic Energy itself functions effectively with the median being these seven energy centre's (Chakras). Everything and everywhere constitutes seven in some respect or the other. For instance, seven seas, seven musical notes (swaraas), seven colours', seven births, seven Rishis (sages), seven powers of motherhood and seven stages of growth, to name a few.

The seven energy centres are considered vital as a person's characteristics, mental set-up and physical ailment can be easily comprehended by studying these seven chakras. Further, a scan of these energy centres will reveal his present state of mind, whether he is going through a rough patch in his personal and professional ends or whether there is a proper flow of energy in his body or not. But improper knowledge of cosmic energy therapy and misusing it on others is not advisable.

I happened to scan a student and revealed to his great shock that he has a problem in his kidneys, the reason being that some people need an extra bit of shock treatment to adopt cosmic energy therapy, which they should understand is only for their good.

6.5. The Chart of Chakras

Based and conceived on the concept of Vedas, this chart of Chakras is the backbone of the Reiki technique. A proper adoption and implementation of the various Chakras characteristics, the presiding deities, incantations, its powers and the organs associated with each chakra are dealt with elaborately in the charts given in Appendix. For instance, to strengthen the energy centre of Visuddhi, proper recitation of the respective deity's incantation can be effectively observed, so much so, the chart can be verified to strengthen any chakra found to be malfunctioning.

The colour of each chakra given in the chart can also be meditated upon for effective results or a pyramid/crystal of the same colour can be used, the details being dealt within a separate chapter.

6.6. Scanning Techniques

With the unfolding of the centres of energy (chakras) to the maximum during the practice of cosmic energy therapy, the practitioner's psychic and sensitivity powers grow. Hence the chakras on our hands can comfortably identify where exactly the patient needs the energy to be transferred to.

Keeping the hand approximately one to four inches away from the patient's body will help you scan the body from head to toe. Then it becomes imperative to understand the difference in the vibration produced in the palms when passing through different parts.

When I was treating some patients along with my students in a Malaysian temple, a 40 year old man came for treatment. A mere look at him suggested he was a chain smoker and I advised him to reduce the habit considerably. Hearing this, one of my students was taken aback. He surprisingly asked me how was it possible for me to decipher his state even without offering him touch therapy or scanning. I just replied that it was a matter of commonsense. That person's odour of cigarette could be smelled even from a distance. That was all. This phenomenon is so widespread nowadays. As Voltaire once observed: "Commonsense is not so common today." How true. We fail to apply commonsense and try to approach everything analytically and intellectually.

When a patient's particular part of the body is cold or if the flow of energy is not smooth, it becomes vital to use the cosmic energy on these areas. Placing both the hands on that part, the cosmic energy can be transferred there.

6.7. Avoid Lips Speaking Contrary to Hearts

The aura surrounding the person differs according to the state of mind he is in. For instance, an angry person reflects a different aura. Sometimes, without any reason, we may feel disinclined to even see a person's face. The aura might be the reason behind this. Similarly it is true that we face failure in every attempt on a particular day if we start the day in the face of unwanted or negatively vibrated person. How true is the proverb "Smile in the lips, poison in the heart." The person might succeed in concealing his vengeance on you with a false smile on his lips, but the aura cannot be hidden and can be easily identified.

6.8. Characteristics of Cosmic Energy

Initially, it is the characteristic of cosmic energy therapy that the healer experiences the patient's pain in him, but soon the pain ceases to exist. A mere glance and a check-up can throw light on the afflicted area and the intensity of pain the patient experiences. To the question of how the hand gets heated up during the therapy, the answer is simple. Cosmic energy channelises into the body through the hand only to make changes. The tissues are attracted to each other and hence the heat. You may have noticed that some people's hands are warmer than those of others.

If the hands are cool, it means that there is no sufficient flow of energy there and this can be rectified by passing more energy into it. Once this is done, a bank of energy is created to bring absolute happiness and health. Another symptom that cosmic energy is at its best is during the transformation. The person either feels fatigued or falls asleep.

6.9. Kirlian Photography

The latest arrival in Kirlian photography can photograph the aura. A costly affair, the method captures the change of mood and the consequent aura produced by it. Though it is not practically possible to photograph whenever the mood changes, still people don't believe what I advocate. They approach the Kirlian photography centres to get them photographed. It merely depicts the state of mood the person was in when he was photographed. It does not remain constant, it changes to the mood. Another irony is these Kirlian photographers also sell crystals deceiving the customers to buy one if they desire to have a positive aura. Kirlian photography costs Rs.100 while a crystal costs Rs.3000. How childish!

6.10. Hand is the Medium of Cosmic Energy

Hands, the instruments of cosmic therapy, can be used to scan the entire body. Though the patients reveal their problems to us, we still scan their bodies to find out if there are any untold problems or problems of psychological nature. After clear analysis, we start the treatment. A master of cosmic therapy should be well equipped with these scanning methods as at all times it is not necessary that the afflicted parts have their source in the same part itself, it may be elsewhere also but the patient may be ignorant of it.

6.11. Pendulum

Pendulum can be effectively used to ascertain the proper functioning of the body centres of energy (chakras). When the pendulum rotates clockwise, the energy centres are sound, but when it goes anticlockwise, learn that a particular part is blocked. Further if the pendulum stops without any movement it implies that a severe block is present in that part. The diameter of the revolution is important as a 6 inch diameter revolution denotes a healthy body and anything below that indicates the intensity of the blockade.

Masters deserve 14 inches to 3 feet diameter as it means that the larger and wider the aura the more they will be effective to that distance. During Reiki treatment, it is this aura that is increased and an increased aura casts a net from afflictions and enhances health.

6.12. In Conversation with the Spirit?

Nearly 90% of people have blocks in the heart's energy centre. And during the therapy, this heaviness is eased considerably. In Chennai, I was able to pinpoint the afflictions of 4 persons after the initiation was over. Stumped by this sudden disclosure of facts, one of the students, a girl, openly asked me whether I seek help from the spirits to be able to tell so accurately. I explained that it is only the energy vibration that reveals all these, and no spirits are involved. Only then was she convinced.

6.13. Self-Scanning

It is mandatory for each one of us to adopt self-scanning and usher in cosmic energy in every part of our body. And it should be understood that a severe blockade is present if more energy passes to a particular spot.

In particular, this self-scanning is helpful to mothers in diagnosing tumours in the breasts and wombs. Early diagnosis helps it to be cured without pain while an unnoticed tumour can become canceric and demand a surgery. The women should shun unwanted fears and come out with these problems if anything occurs at an early stage which otherwise, would only lead to unwanted surgeries. Adopt self-scanning and be healthy.

Chapter 13: Aura/ Magnetic Field

The Sun Light and Aura

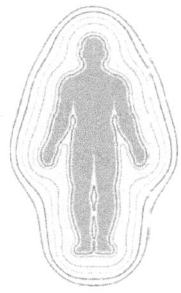

How is magnetic field related to Past Lives?

We all have seen pictures and paintings of God's across various traditions but one thing that is common among all of them is the circle of light around their head. This circle of light not only surrounds the head, it also extends all around the body it is known as the Aura /magnetic field. The aura is part of our energy body that extends around the physical body.

The aura is electromagnetic energy field that extends all around our body for about 4-5feet (in an average healthy body). In science this is called as the bio field.

Everything in this universe has an aura. If we study ancient Indian texts especially the yoga sutras we will come to know the fine anatomy of human chakra system which is actually a very important aspect of our Aura. Aura represents our physical, mental, emotional as well as spiritual energies. Aura can reveal a lot of unsaid information about us, our innermost desires, feelings, emotions etc.

The aura is energy field that surrounds and interpenetrates the physical body, it also process and relay information from universe to our physical body. As per research and ancient texts the aura has 7 layers.

Nowadays Hi-tech electronic gadgets and instruments can detect the fine subtle vibrations in our surroundings; it has become possible for us to capture a glimpse of the human aura by the help of Kirlian camera or PIP (Poly contrast interference photography), DAS (Digital Aura Scanning system), RFI (Resonant Field Imaging) etc.

The Sun Light and Aura

The Vedas assert Sun (Surya) to be the creator of the material universe (Prakruthi). The Rig-Veda, mentions Surya with particular reverence for the "rising sun" and its symbolism as dispeller of darkness, one who empowers knowledge and complete life.

Sun is the ultimate source of energy on this lively planet – THE EARTH. The life force exists on this planet due to the optimum temperature maintained by the Earth.

Nowadays we are bombarded with paranoid messages about how dangerous the sun light is. In this busy life style sometimes for months we are not in the sun and many people think that it's dangerous to expose skin to sunlight, but sun rays are very essential to every living being. Solar energy is the best energy to keep us fit and fine. Sun rays cleanse the Aura and easily penetrate positive energy to the physical body. An early morning and evening walk in mild sun rays is always beneficial.

Ancient yogis and many other cultures around the world knew how to use the sun energy to heal any kind of illness and bring back radiant health. Ancient Greeks have history of using sunlight as a form of healing therapy. This was called heliosis. Now, sunlight therapy is called as heliotherapy.

Here are benefits of getting a moderate amount of sun exposure:

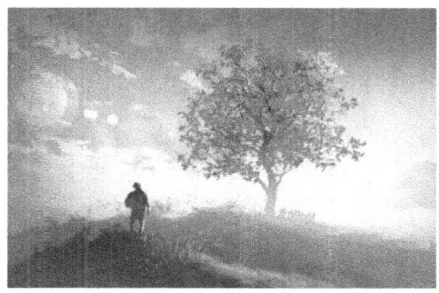

Huge amount of vitamin D

Cure's depression

Promotes bone health

Supports immune system

Protects against memory loss

Good for loosing excess fat

Strengthens teeth

Kills bad bacteria

Heals skin disorders

Lowers cholesterol

Lowers blood pressure

Cleanses the blood and blood vessels

Increases oxygen content in blood

Works as anti-cancer agent

How is magnetic field [Aura] related to Past Lives?

We are multi-dimensional spirit beings; the Aura is the living template, it stores all energy and information throughout our life. When we die, we move out of the physical body but the Aura continues the journey. Although we take rebirth and a new body, the Aura remains the same. It carries all the experiences [emotional and mental] as well as, all the knowledge and information we have gained through many lifetimes.

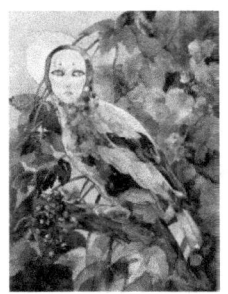

Whatever we see, observe or feel will be recorded in our aura. It has the link with the Akashic records, because of which we can retain information of who and what we have been in other lives.

Past Life Regression therapy can be a very useful way to work through, any unsolved physical, emotional or spiritual questions/problems. A troublesome past life, behaves much like unresolved early childhood trauma affecting the life of the adult.

Past life regression works on the body, mind, emotions, and spirit. Its chief purpose is to make our life easier, better and more fulfilling. It addresses the root cause and enables deep change to take place at the very source of the problem. It does not deal with external symptoms. It directly addresses the internal cause.

Our past will always have an effect on our present and future. Anything related to past, a past desire, a past thought, past feeling, a past emotion, a past promise, a past decision or a past traumatic experience can be cleared through past life regression.

Past life regression helps individuals to understand the karmic patterns involved and the resultant energy blockages. It helps to overcome phobias, improves relationships by helping the person to understand the past life relationship with the particular individual or group of people. Until this is understood, clashes and friction in one's present life relation is inevitable. Once the understanding flows, the person will be able to see the larger perspective and therefore the relationships are improved or 'healed'.

Past life regression helps us to explore our past lives and through this exploration we realize that we are eternal beings. This removes the fear of death for once and all.

Chapter 14: The Sixth Chakra

The sixth chakra is also called the light chakra and can be located directly in between your eyes. It deals with insight and acceptance of the unearthly, the supernatural, and the unexplainable. It is often blocked by the illusions individuals set up for themselves.

The light chakra and the third eye

Many people associate an open, healthy sixth chakra to an open third eye. This is because, once the other five chakras are kept open and healthy, you will soon realize that the physical boundaries and laws of this world can be transcended. You will soon see and learn about the spirits that surround us, teach us, and try to clear a path for us so that we, too, will become one with our perfect, higher selves.

Now, some people fear the third eye, particularly because the third eye allows people to see things and entities that have been disregarded by the common population as myths and mere stories. But you must not be afraid. The strongest illusion people make up for themselves is the illusion of separation. The sixth chakra will teach you that nothing is isolated, and that everything is connected. Therefore, even the strange spirits and the unfamiliar entities that share this world with our physical bodies, are connected to us. You must not be afraid of this, as fear is but another illusion.

Opening the sixth chakra

Follow the steps detailed below to open your light chakra.

Step 1: Find a quiet place where you can sit, undisturbed.

Step 2: Clear your mind. Breathe slowly, surely and deeply. Release all your inhibitions and fears. Remember that to be truly in tune with yourself and the universe, you must open this vital chakra and align it with the others.

Step 3: Now think of all the illusions you have made yourself believe. Think of the illusion of separation, and focus on the truth of interconnectedness. Feel all the elements in the room, all the individuals who are within your proximity radiate and exchange energy with you. Even the plants and the animals are part of this world, and so they are part of you. Let their energy flow to and from you.

Step 4: Acknowledge that there are other entities in this world, and the other worlds your physical cannot visit. Do not let fear cloud your judgment, or skepticism prevent a deeper understanding. Instead, embrace that which you cannot understand, and rest assured in the knowledge, that you are connected to them, as they are connected to you.

Step 5: Imagine your sixth chakra glowing faintly in between your eyes. Slowly open it to the energy of all that is around you. Let the energy of your environment recharge your sixth chakra, and help your eyes see clearer.

Note that not everyone is able to successfully open their third eyes. This takes practice and constant meditation.

You can also recharge and strengthen your sixth chakra by wearing or keeping anything of the color indigo. Eat blackberries, blueberries and drink red wine or grape juice to keep your sixth chakra energized.

Chapter 15: Meditation

Meditation is certainly an old art as it goes back to around 5000 years where an Indian text named Malini Vijaya Tantra talks about it.

While talking about yoga, we can't ignore the contributions of meditation in making yoga practice effective. Where yoga relaxes the body, meditation is a process of relaxing the mind. Meditation is a part of yoga; when a proper balance is struck between them, you get to attain the state where there is only calmness, positive vibration and inner peace.

Here, technically meditation is a conscious effort taken to calm ourselves. Human mind keeps working all the time and thinks non-stop. With the help of meditation we can remove clutters out of our mind by concentrating on our breathing tune and at the end of it you think nothing.

Meditation has been followed for a long time. Initially it was a tool to attain a spiritual height, but now in this modern era it has become the most important means to relax, rejuvenate ourselves. Being a tool for stress management as well it helps in giving a proper balance between the mental, emotional and physical scales of the person.

How to meditate

☐ Sit in a comfortable pose/asana (preferably in padmasana on the floor).

☐ However you sit, make sure the spine is straight and head up. Mind and body are interlinked, so if you dip your mind will go out of balance.

☐ Now look straight, close your eyes and imagine you are on the top of the sky.

- You can also keep the eyes open as they help in keeping you at present.

- Now slowly concentrate on the breathing movement and fall in its tune.

- You can start counting your breath slowly in your mind, or chant some mantra softly

- When the thoughts wander away, slowly without a jerk bring them back to the starting point by concentrating on the breath.

- Do not stop yourself, just be calm and relaxed.

- It is difficult to concentrate when one is on a high on emotion.

- Find a nice place to sit and meditate, as place plays an important role in effective meditation. A calm, silent place with fewer disturbances will suffice.

☐ Initially the length of mediation can be around 7-10 minutes and extend to 30 minutes.

Benefits of meditation

☐ The benefit of meditation can be obtained only when it is practiced on a daily basis. A routine in meditation can make the whole experience wonderful.

☐ It increases our concentration and clarity.

☐ It helps in stress management and anxiety reduction.

☐ It strengthens our emotional stability.

☐ This helps in gaining a sharp mind and thereby improving our perfection.

☐ It is highly beneficial if followed during pregnancy.

☐ This increases the mental strength and gives the physical body the support to effectively performance.

Chapter 16: Timeout: How to Perform a Quick Healing Session

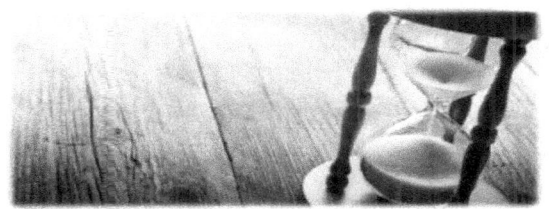

It's not always possible to do a full healing session. In times like these, we'd better make good use of the time we have available.

Here's a suggestion on how to conduct a quick treatment. It's an abridged version of the full treatment. Enjoy!

Have the patient sit on a chair, legs and arms uncrossed. This is because the uncrossed is an open position, making it easier to receive energy, as opposed e.g. to the closed positions such as lotus etc.

Hands on shoulders.

Hands on the head.

One hand on the upper neck, and the other on the forehead.

One hand on the back of the neck, and the other between the throat and heart chakras.

One hand on the breast bone, the other on the back, mirrored.

One hand on the solar plexus, the other on the back, mirrored.

One hand on the lower stomach, the other on the back, mirrored.

Ground them by placing both hands on their feet for about a minute.

Above are the basic steps. Spend 2-3 minutes in each position, unless you are guided otherwise. Below are some things to be aware of throughout the treatment:

Take it easy, don't rush. Patients can sense these things.

If you or the patient are uncomfortable touching certain areas, keep your hands slightly away from the body, in the aura.

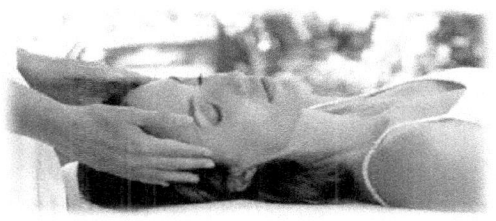

Remember to offer your patient some water at the end of the session.

Explaining What a Reiki Practitioner Does

By Taryn Walker

It's a common question. "So what do you do?" Honestly it has always driven me nuts and I have been a little facetious at times and said things like "Oh you know, I eat, I sleep, I go swimming and sometimes I enjoy long walks in the mountains". Sorry! But I know that usually what people are actually asking is "What do you do for a living?" "How do you make money?" "What's your purpose?"

When I made the switch from English teacher to Reiki practitioner I noticed quite a difference in the way people responded to what I do. "I'm a Reiki practitioner" is often met with an awkward silence followed by an "Oh". I only realised just how misunderstood and misrepresented Reiki is once I started practicing and teaching it professionally. There's a lot of hogwash on the Internet and it's given Reiki a bad name. So it got me thinking. How can I present what I do without using the word Reiki? And wouldn't it be nice if everyone expressed what they did for a living in a way that made people understand what they actually do as opposed to what they're called.

So what do I do?

"I help people to move towards balance and wholeness by using a simple relaxation technique which activates the body's natural healing response".

That sounds awesome. I'd try that.

"I guide people to reconnect with their inner magic".

I'm intrigued. I'd like to know more!

"I help people to realise that they are so much more than a physical body. As they begin to understand themselves as multi-layered beings a beautiful journey inwards begins and this depth of experience brings great meaning and purpose to life".

Wow! That sounds incredible. How do you do that?

As you can see there are so many ways to present your profession and it can be enjoyable to be creative in your explanations. Conversations about what we do can be really interesting.

So instead of being rigidly identified with the name of your profession -Reiki Master, Finance Manager, Accountant, Housewife - why not try and describe how you help. What you do is valuable in so many ways if you really think about it.

Be passionate in your sharing. Be proud of how you contribute, no matter how small you think that is. People respond well to passion because it is authentic. As a Reiki practitioner and teacher I have found this to be a wonderful way of letting others know just how much I love Reiki and what people can achieve through regular Reiki practice.

How would you describe what you do without mentioning your job title? Do you practice Reiki for a living? How would you explain what you do without using the word Reiki? Why not share your descriptions below to spread some ideas around our community? Your enthusiasm may even be contagious!

Explaining Reiki to Others

By Angie Webster

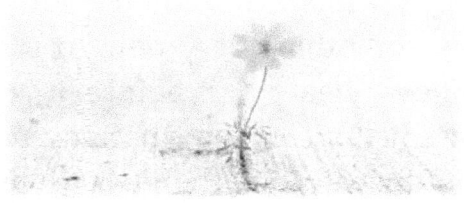

One of the most interesting challenges I have met as a Reiki practitioner has been learning how to explain what Reiki is and the ways it works to help us to those who know little or nothing about Reiki. I find that a different explanation is needed depending upon the person to whom you are speaking.

Some people are ready to learn more than others, so it is best to tailor the explanation to the needs of the specific person. Many people will want to learn more as they take in a small amount of information, whereas if you overload them with too much information at once, they may lose interest or misunderstand something. Think of when you are explaining something very new to a child who has never heard of it before. It is best to give a small bit of information and let them lead the way with their questions.

It may be easiest for you to think back to your own level of understanding when you first heard of Reiki. What sort of things did you wonder about? What information did you find confusing? What information did you find helpful? When I first the word Reiki years ago, I was very confused about how to pronounce it (RAY-key) and what it did. I decided it wasn't for me based on a few pieces of unclear information. This can be the case for many people, so go slow and easy. It is not going to be helpful information if you overwhelm the person and they may become confused.

The best way I have found to explain Reiki is to say that it is an energy healing method that is usually done by placing the hands in a series of positions over or slightly above the body. If the person wants to know more, I will explain that Reiki promotes healing by activating the relaxation response and helping the body to balance itself from a very deep level.

Sometimes it is best to offer a demonstration of Reiki, if the person is open to that. The experience of Reiki says more than words ever could.

Something that can frighten people who are new to learning about Reiki is the use of spiritual terminology. This kind of terminology can lead to the fear that Reiki is a religious practice or that it goes against certain religions. It can also lead to thoughts that Reiki is ineffective. Many people are uncomfortable with the word "spiritual" or "spirit". Use your best judgment in deciding if the person is able to understand that healing occurs on all levels, including the soul or spirit level.

Some people will want you to explain how Reiki works. No one really knows the answer to this. But you can tell them that Reiki allows positive energy to flow into the body through the hands of the practitioner and that this balances and heals the energy in the body. You could also explain some of the things that Reiki has been scientifically shown to do, such as decrease pain levels, speed healing and relax the mind and body. Make sure that the person understands that Reiki can only do good and can never cause harm.

Let your own understanding of the person you are speaking to guide you in what to say. When a person wants to know more and is enthusiastic, you will sense that. Likewise, you will learn to sense when a person is not able to take in too much information. Remember, it is not your role to force information onto someone who is not ready to receive it. Allow time and patience and be at peace. When the person is ready to receive more information about Reiki, they will know it is time. As healers, part of the process is allowing things to go forward at the pace that is comfortable to each individual. And acceptance that each of our paths is different.

CHAPTER 17: CHAKRAS AND AURA

Why do we need to know energy systems?

There are different energy systems. In order to do Reiki, all we need to know is where the 7 main chakras (energy centres) are located and possibly different parts of the body. These 7 chakras are shown in the diagram below.

This is because as Reiki Healers we won't be diagnosing or treating patients – just channeling healing to them. This is the same as Mikao Usui's original Reiki practices (it was Dr. Hayashi who introduced medical elements). We are not doctors and it would not be professional to do this.

What are energy systems?

This is the general information that you need to know about different energy systems. There are similarities between each system. These similarities are:

There are main energy centres (7 chakras or gates or drops).

There is a grid of meridians, channels or lines and on the body is crystalised onto those meridians.

Finally, energy, or chi, can be divided into approx 2 or 3 elements (depending on different cultural interpretations).

DIAGRAM OF AURA AND LAYERS

DIAGRAM: CHAKRAS AND AURA

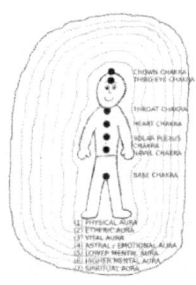

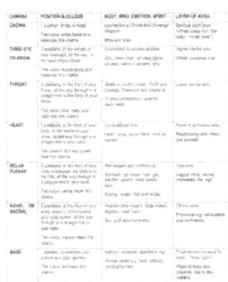

FURTHER BACKGROUND INFORMATION FOR ADVANCED STUDENTS ONLY

If you would like to find out more, I have written some background information below. There have also been many books written on this. If you find this confusing, it is not necessary to know this and you can skip the next section.

CHAKRAS (ancient yoga sutras India)

The body has numerous chakras and energy meridians. However, there are 7 major chakras and 21 minor chakras. These are said to be "psychic" energy centres, rather than physical places. Practices such as Acupuncture, Acupressure, Reflexology and Shiatsu work with these many different chakras and meridians. The major chakras are connected to a channel in the spine (which is why you need a straight back during Reiki and Meditation). In Reiki, we concentrate on the 7 major chakras (although healing is sent throughout the entire body and aura).

CHINESE ENERGY SYSTEM (CHI, MERIDIANS AND GATES)

In Chinese, energy ("Chi") is divided into 2 parts: Yin and Yang. When we are ill or unhappy, these two parts are not in balance and harmony. There are also 12 meridians and 5 elements (earth, water, fire, wood, metal). There are also gates instead of chakras.

For more information on Chinese and Japanese Energy Systems: "Spirit of Reiki" by Walter Lubeck, Frank Arjava Petter, William Rand.

JAPANESE ENERGY SYSTEM (KI)

In the Japanese energy system, there are 7 types of Ki energy. This is taken from William Lubeck's article.

KEKKI — this is energy of the blood. It is the lowest energy, the basic foundation energy. It gives strength and power. Connected to the Root Chakra.

SHIOKE - is mineral energy. It is concerned with bodily function and organizes the Kekki. Also connected to the Root Chakra.

MIZUKE — is water energy. Enables relationship and communication. It is the basic energy of all emotions, and allows for nourishment and metabolism. Connected with the Sacral Chakra.

KUKI — is air or gas energy. Enables self-discovery, logic, harmony and free will. Related to the Solar Plexus Chakra.

DENKI — the energy of thunder. Enables balance between our own needs and ego, and others. Also associated with love, ethics and our relationship with the Divine. Connected with the Heart Chakra.

JIKI – "magnetic power" or "gathering force". It manages the lower 5 energies and also enables truth and insight. Associated with the Throat Chakra.

REIKI – is the energy of soul or spirit. It is the highest energy and manages the lower energies. It is also linked with the Divine and connects Divine to material energies. Associated with the Brow Chakra.

DIVINE ENERGY OR SHINKI – there is also Divine energy. This is the combination of all the types of energy. It is where energy begins and ends. It is associated with the

Crown Chakra but works outside of the body.

However, "Reiki healing" is concerned with the whole system of the body, mind, emotions and spirit (i.e. different from Reiki Ki, energy type).

AYURVEDIC ENERGY SYSTEM (3 BODY ELEMENTS)

Ayurveda means "science of life" in Sanskrit and is at least 5000 years old. In Ayurveda and Ayurvedic Reiki, disease is due to an imbalance of 3 energies of the body (3 doshas: Vata, Pitta and Kapha). A person has all 3 vital energies, but one (or two) energies will be more prominent, making that person a particular energy type e.g. a Vata type.

VATA – Primary element is air. A Vata person is

PITTA – Primary element is fire. A Pitta person is pale and freckly.

KAPHA – Primary element is water. A Kapha person is

The universe also has 5 elements (Panch Maha Bhootas). These are 5 types of energy which are also inside the body: space (ether), Vaayu (air), Agni (fire) Ap (water), Prithvi (earth). There are 7 types of tissue in the body: plasma and lymph, blood, muscle, fat, bone, bone marrow and nerve tissue, reproductive tissue.

KUNDALINI ENERGY SYSTEM (14 NADIS)

In Kundalini, there are 7 main chakras and 14 Nadis (a network of channels). The most important are Ida, Pingala and Sushumna.

PINGALA - is the right channel (right nostril) and is red, masculine, hot and links to the sun.

IDA - is the left channel (left nostril) and is white, feminine, cool and links to the moon.

SUSHUMNA - is the central channel where kundalini energy flows along our spine up to our crown.

MULADHARA - these three energies meet at Muladhara (Yukta Triveni).

IT IS IMPORTANT not to raise the Kundalini energy too soon as it will be too powerful and will affect your well-being. Take your time with any energy or spiritual work. This is one reason why you need a teacher and guidance.

TIBETAN ENERGY SYSTEM

(DROPS, 5 KOSAs, 4 ELEMENTS, WINDS)

This is by Lama Govinda in Foundations of Tibetan Mysticism. There are 7 chakras (drops). In Tibetan, the energy that flows through us is called Lung (aka Prana, Chi, Ki).

There are also 5 energy layers called 5 sheaths (kosa)

1. PHYSICAL BODY (anna-maya-kosa) – Gross (internal organs) and Less Gross (external e.g. skin).

2. SUBTLE BODY (prana-maya-kosa) – The energy channels or winds.

3. THOUGHT OR PERSONALITY BODY (mano-maya-kosa) – Thoughts and mental processes. Connects to physical body.

4. BODY OF POTENTIAL CONSCIOUSNESS (vijnana-maya-kosa) – Connection with the universe, Buddha.

5. BODY OF BLISS OR SAMBHOGAKAYA (ananda-maya-kosa) – the highest universal consciousness, enlightenment.

There are also 4 elements to the body: water (feeling aggregates, and fluids), earth (solidity, physical aggregates), fire (discrimination/logic) and air/wind (conversational/communication).

Energy is called Winds.

AURA

AURA (SPIRITUAL ENERGY SYSTEM OUTSIDE BODY)

Your aura is the energy field around your body. There are 7 layers of the aura, starting from your body, and moving outwards. Your aura can be different colours, shapes and sizes, depending upon your personality, thoughts, emotions and well-being. Imbalances (which may lead to illness) can show in your aura, before they manifest in your body and mind.

1. PHYSICAL AURA - physical body and practical, day to day matters. This is the

layer closest to the body (inner layer) and is the layer that people sometimes see. Relates to base chakra.

2. ETHERIC AURA - emotional e.g. self-esteem and confidence. Relates to navel chakra.

3. VITAL AURA - logical mind, mental processes, the 'ego'. Relates to solar plexus chakra.

4. ASTRAL OR EMOTIONAL AURA - relationship with others and yourself. Relates to heart chakra.

5. LOWER MENTAL AURA - inner wisdom. Relates to throat chakra.

6. HIGHER MENTAL AURA - Divine, universal love. Relates to third eye chakra.

7. SPIRITUAL AURA - intuition, Divine Wisdom. This is the layer furthest away from the body (outer layer). Relates to crown chakra.

AURIC/ESOTERIC CHAKRAS

As well as the 7 major chakras, some energy and Reiki schools (e.g. Celtic Reiki) say that there are additional chakras outside of your body.

Below you there is an "Earth Star Chakra", then a "Gala Gateway". Above you, there is a "Soul Star Chakra", then a "Stellar Gateway", and then 352 levels above you to the source of the energy.

There are also other chakras within your aura: "Sacred Heart", "Etheric Heart", "Higher Heart, "Hara" and "Causal Body".

CHAKRA AND ENERGY SUMMARY

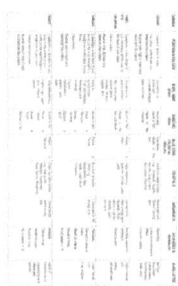

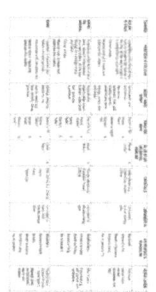

For more information on Japanese Ki, see Walter Lubeck founder of Rainbow Reiki.

Different Reiki schools use crystals, for example Celtic Reiki.

Chapter 18: The History Of Reiki

What Is Reiki?

Reiki is universal energy and also the name of the healing art that uses this healing energy for positive change. There is no direct translation from Japanese, however loosely Rei means spiritual, higher power or creator and Ki means vital energy or life force. Reiki is not associated with a particular religion or practice.

It is difficult to describe Reiki to those who have never experienced it. Just like it would be difficult to describe the sun to someone who has never ventured out of a dark cave. Reiki can be described like the sun's energy. You can feel its warmth on your body. You can feel it on your skin and to your core. It provides plants with food through photosynthesis. Through the vital energy in the plants, animals receive nourishment. The sun provides animals (and humans) with vitamin d. It provides healing and nourishment. Yet you cannot see all the ways the sun is working to give life and heal. However, the sun is there, and accessible to all. In this way, Reiki energy is there and accessible. You can feel it, it flows into you, and through you to heal and nourish. Many people describe receiving Reiki as a gentle warmth flowing into them. Most people describe feeling a deep relaxation.

Reiki flows into us from the universal source and goes where it is needed and how it is needed. How you experience that flow is an individual experience. It can vary each time depending on what you are being treated for, the practitioner treating you, and your own current emotional, mental, and physical state.

As a practitioner, (anyone who has received a Reiki attunement is a practitioner) Reiki can enter your body through two different routes. Some believe it is pulled through the feet, from the earth's energy. Others believe it is pulled from above, through the crown or top of your head. Wherever you feel Reiki entering you as a practitioner, know that the supply is limitless, and when healing, it is not your own ki being used or depleted, but the infinite supply of ki coming from the universe to heal you and the recipient. Reiki heals both the recipient and the practitioner – each and every time. This is why it is beneficial to give Reiki treatments to others – when you give Reiki, it flows through and out your body and removes your blockages and heals you as well.

In giving a Reiki treatment to yourself or another, the Reiki energy flows from the palms of your hands into the recipient. The energy flows smoothly, varying in speed, intensity, temperature, and sensation depending on the illness, emotional state, blockages, personal energy, and willingness to accept change and healing.

No one knows why Reiki works, or even exactly how it works. It is currently beyond the knowledge of science and human understanding. However, we know, based on medical studies, anecdotes, and personal experience that Reiki **does** work. Likewise, it has been found that a person does not need to believe in Reiki to experience its benefits, Or in the case of some studies, even know that they are receiving Reiki (vs placebo) to experience beneficial healing. We don't need to understand Reiki to know that it has value.

What Can Reiki Do?

Reiki energy can boost your well-being and your vital life force/ki.

Reiki can treat pain or unease associated with disease.

Reiki can remove stagnant energy blockages.

Reiki can reduce stress, reduce blood pressure, slow heart rate, and lower cortisol (stress hormone) levels.

Reiki can heal past and present emotional trauma and psychological pain.

Reiki can improve your immune system.

Reiki can boost your body's natural healing abilities.

Reiki can act as a complimentary treatment to traditional medicine.

Reiki can add vitality and wellness to your life.

Reiki can aid in giving self-compassion, love, and healing to yourself and others.

Reiki can be easily accessed and used anywhere, anytime.

How Does Reiki Heal?

The human body is a complex, beautiful system of organs, tissues, cells, blood, bone, and more, all working together in concert. Yet, the human being is much more than a physical entity. We are much more than blood and bone. We are the ebb and flow of energy, of spirit, of emotion, of ki – the vital life force that is a part of every living thing.

Traditional medicine focuses on the physical aspect of health. The final sickness, symptom, or disease. However, the disease is the last stop in the continuum, and traditional medicine (looking at the physical) treats the body – not the disruption of ki that led the physical body down the road toward disharmony and dis-ease.

The disruption of ki leads to disharmony, stagnation, and blockages in the human energy field (addressed throughout time and culture as chakras, meridians, aura, spirit, subconscious, energy, etc.) — these disruptions, over time, precictably lead to disease. However, by practicing Reiki, and by addressing disruption in the ki, we can heal by focusing on the beginning or root of dis-ease. We can even prevent illness by removing the discordance before sickness develops.

Medical science has even noted the phenomenon that major life stressors can predict your likelihood of becoming ill. The Holmes and Rahe Stress Scale (1967) has a list of 43 life events over the previous 2 years of a person's life. You tabulate the number of events and the weighted value of the events to determine how likely it is that you will develop a major illness within the near future. Traditional medicine recognizes that stress, emotional trauma, and psychological pain (causing a disruption in ki) make it more likely that a person will become ill in the near future —

however, they do not have an easily accessible healing modality to prevent that illness from occurring. Rather, they say – "yes, you are more likely to get sick – come to us when you do and we'll treat you".

Reiki on the other hand, treats the ki disruption before it results in illness. Or, if you are coming to Reiki after a health problem occurs, it addresses the root cause, the flow, or blockage of energy.

Some of the life stressors included in the stress scale are: death of a spouse, divorce, marital separation, personal injury, jail, marriage, termination of employment, pregnancy, change in financial status, taking out a mortgage or loan, change in personal habits, vacation, change in dietary habits, and more. If you know that life stressors can lead to illness, know also that you can use Reiki to heal and encourage health so that these stressors do not lead to disease.

Using Reiki To Heal

To use Reiki to heal you can either seek out the services of a Reiki practitioner or receive a Reiki attunement and practice self-healing. After a few short hours in a Reiki Level 1 course you will be able to receive and give Reiki healing energy. In the next chapter, we'll discuss the Reiki attunement process, the levels of Reiki practice, and choosing a Reiki Master.

As mentioned before, you can use Reiki for emotional, mental, spiritual and physical healing.

Dr. Usui, the founder of Reiki, searched for a method that would heal both the body and the spirit, and not drain the practitioner's own energy. He found this in Reiki. By passing down the attunement to

Reiki energy, we are also able to access Reiki.

When Dr. Usui was first practicing medicine, he worked with beggars on the streets. He healed their physical wounds so that they could go on to work and live more productive lives. However, he found that the people he healed would frequently return to the street to beg. He asked them why, and they said it was easier to beg on the street than to change their pattern and move into a new life. He realized that he had healed the physical body, but not the emotional and spiritual body. He developed Reiki to help heal all three. Many times, especially in the case of chronic illness and stress related illness, a healing is not complete unless it addresses both the physical and emotional aspects of dis-ease.

Don't focus only on physical symptoms when you are using Reiki to heal. For a person to be fully healed, their psychological, emotional, and physical health must all be taken into account.

If possible, use Reiki self-healing on yourself every day. You can practice it while watching tv, while reading, while lying in bed before getting up in the morning, or whenever you have a spare moment. It is not necessary to concentrate only on healing – you must merely set the intention to act as a conduit for Reiki and to let it heal.

When treating another, you may want to treat them more frequently in the beginning stages: whether daily or multiple times a week, and then space the treatments out to once a week, once a month, or less. Each person will have a different need.

Although, when giving Reiki, you also receive Reiki, it is a best practice to give yourself self-treatments, and even, receive treatments from other Reiki practitioners. The purpose is to keep your energy flowing, your ki in a state of openness and balance, and your body, mind, and spirit healthy.

Dr. Usui gave us a daily mantra to keep us in good health. It is known as the five principles of Reiki. An indirect translation follows.

Dr. Usui's Secret To Happiness And Health

Just for today,

Do not be angry, do not worry,

Be grateful and work hard,

Be kind to others,

Every morning and every evening join your hands in prayer

And remember these words

As a Reiki practitioner, say these words to yourself every day. You don't have to promise not to be angry for the rest of forever – just for today. You don't have to promise not to worry for the rest of forever – just for today. Practice gratitude and devote yourself to fulfilling your life's purpose through your work. Always be kind to others. Meditate and pray on this every day.

This, and the practice of Reiki, is Dr. Usui's secret to happiness and health.

Key Take Away

Reiki is a gentle, yet powerful healing system developed in Japan by a Zen Buddhist monk named Mikao Usui. It is a form of touch, or energy healing that is natural, easy to use, and available to everyone. The healing energy used in Reiki is passed down from teacher to student in an attunement process. The attunement opens students up to the Reiki energy:

Usui attuned his students to Reiki and his students then attuned their students — resulting in the long and vast lineage of Reiki we have today.

Reiki heals physical, spiritual, and psychological wounds — the entire human being. Reiki focuses on healing the root of disease/disharmony at an energetic level instead of only treating physical symptoms.

Chapter 19: Receiving Angelic Reiki

Synopsis

We have taken a look at how to perform Angelic Reiki... but how do we receive it?

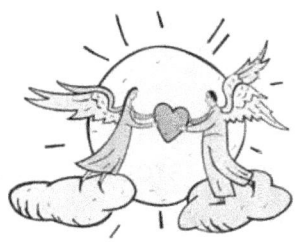

Learning To Be Open

Giving and getting are yin and yang, the counterpart of the infinity symbol—looping backward and forward, neither side bigger than the other, both built-in to the larger whole.

Many of us need to learn how to get into a place of comfortable receiving, slowly, one baby step at a time. I get a compliment with a simple thank you , regardless that inside you are discounting the words.

This is an acquired skill. You can learn this. You can let the words and more importantly your healing sink in and fill your empty spaces. You can accept a gift with a thank you and let that be adequate, you have to learn to open up to be able to receive.

You can let other people help you with grace and the profound gratitude that somebody or something wishes to be of service. You can be open and can let other people have the fun of giving.

And ultimately, this is how you can give more easily, by learning to refill your needs with receiving.

You also need to learn about giving—that giving to quench your own need will never be adequate.

When you give, not from a complete heart, but from a void space that requires recognition, you will be exhausted. Giving from your own need leads to bitterness, victimhood, and distress.

Here are some reminders to help you learn this new skill.

To begin, you have to accept the basic premise that you are enough—that before you give a thing, before you receive anything, you are enough simply being here. The act of giving or getting doesn't change this in the least.

You have to become more discerning with giving. You have to learn to examine your needs as well as the needs of other people. To see when your gift is really given from love and when it comes with expectations. To see if the expectations are self-imposed and if they come from other people.

You have to make room in your life for receiving. This includes being aware of all the ways you may receive, whether it's accepting kind words, a stranger's grin, or connecting with the Angels. Know that as you receive, you are getting to be more comfortable with the art of receiving. Stay conscious of how your receiving empowers those who are giving to you.

Relax into the feeling of receiving—get to be okay with the feeling of openness that's necessary to really receive. Allow this openness to be available to receive.

Chapter 20: What makes a good healer?

Following the principles of reiki, stated in Chapter 2, is very important to become a good healer. A good healer is someone positive, someone who has pure intent. If you wish to engage on the path of healing, it is important to look after yourself. Most healers start their paths by going through a healing crisis that forces them to heal themselves, often with the help of others. This is nothing to worry about. It's a spring clean of your house. And in order to be a good healer, you need to have your house in order.

You might find that when you discover the incredible power of reiki, you will be so excited that you will want to heal everyone. And then you might fall into the St Bernard syndrome of wanting to do that against the person's will. Or when someone refuses your good deed, you will be offended or think or say something unkind. We have all done that at some point in our lives. Just be aware of this lesson so that you can overcome it. If you don't you might find that the reiki will stop flowing through you.

To put it in a more positive way, you will find that the more you respect the reiki principles, the stronger your healer power will become. What will also improve it is using it as often as possible, but also whilst doing that, to be detached as to the outcome of what you do.

I find that the best way to do this is to start all my healing sessions with a little prayer that goes like this: "I ask all my angels and guides to help me being a pure channel for the divine light and reiki for the highest good of [name of the person] today and in divine timing". I then thank my angels and guides for helping me in that goal.

It is important when you start on your healing path to receive some encouragement. And for that purpose, it is good to get some feedback. The best feedback, however, is unsolicited. And due to the fact that healing continues sometimes for more than forty eight hours after a healing session, you might only get feedback days after the session if not weeks. Patience and trust is needed. And it doesn't matter if you don't feel anything or if your recipient does not feel the energy. Sensations are interesting but they are not necessary to the healing process. You might find however that the more you use reiki, the more sensitive you become. I want to add that it is a side effect and should by no mean become the goal. Clairvoyance is not a sign of a good healer either. In fact contrary to a common belief, clairvoyance is not a sign of spiritual advancement; it is just a sign that the person knows how to use mental energy.

The only thing that really matters is to be non judgmental, to have pure intent and to want to be of service to God and to serve the highest good and interests of the person who comes to you. A good healer is not interested in symptoms but rejoices in the opening of the heart.

In time, you might find that there are people that you cannot work on. It is a sign of strength to recognise this and to be able to refer these people to other healers. Being possessive of your clients is a hinder to your healing power too.

A good healer has gone through the crisis that other experience and has developed the empathy and the understanding of the human heart. It takes quite a few heartaches and experiences to reach that maturity. And even then, you have to be extremely careful not to become dogmatic. Just because you might have gone through cancer does not mean that how you dealt with it will suit all other people who have cancer, nor that you can understand every one who goes through cancer.

A word about the rescuer archetype. Archetypes are personality types that encapsulate a mode of interacting with others. There is an archetype called the rescuer and when you start on the healing path, you should be aware of it. A rescuer is someone whose raison d'être is to help others. She sees things to fix in others but not in herself. She relentlessly helps others and gets from these deeds a meaning for her life. In effect, if you are quite happy and content, she might totally ignore you. Often, however, she will demand in return some sort of allegiance. It might be that she calls the shots. Or that you need to show gratitude a certain way. Or that she takes over part of your life and actually gives you advice or help in areas where you have never asked for. That is not at all the true spirit of healing, nor of reiki. Please question your own motives as to why you want to be a healer? There is nothing wrong with having a rescuer archetype in us, as long as we know it is there and that it can come in the way of our path.

Conclusion

Reiki, as mentioned earlier, is very easy. Reiki healing should be natural and should be performed without any effort. Just lightly and gently place your hands on the right positions to experience Reiki for yourself.

Reiki healing will provide you with the energy that you need so you can deal with negative influences surrounding you and let them go. A lot of people have benefitted from Reiki, since it not only treats the superficial layers of a condition but goes deeply to fix the root of the problem. Reiki is not only able to improve one's self but also the relationships people have with other people. Although a Reiki healer can provide you with the energy that you need, it is still important to keep in mind that the results ultimately depend on you. If you want to reap the benefits of

Reiki, you need to want to help yourself. If, deep inside, you are not making an effort to improve or heal yourself, no matter how many Reiki sessions you take or no matter how many times you self-treat yourself, Reiki will simply just never work.

Unlike other spiritual and traditional healing methods, you should never exert any effort in Reiki treatment. Allow the energy to flow naturally. The purpose of this is to make sure that the energy that flows through uses its own intelligence to guide itself through the body. Once a Reiki master has performed attunement on you, your own healing energy will begin to naturally flow. Just place your hands on yourself or on anyone, even your pet, who needs healing, relaxation or a sense of inner peace. The energy will flow naturally from you and the beneficial and positive effects will soon be felt and seen.

While you may be tempted to start focusing and redirecting energy, it is very important that you remember to relax, as doing so will decrease the optimal flow of energy. The greatest success will only be achieved if you let the energy flow through by itself. Always remind yourself to stay relaxed and isolated from the process and just simply focus on your intent to heal and maintain the flow of energy. It is also important not to judge your experience, whether you were the receiver or the giver. Remember, Reiki is most effective when used mainly to enhance and improve your overall well-being and not as a substitute, especially to conventional, medical treatments. With Reiki, you can always relax and let go of your worries, as there is nothing you can do that may go wrong.

www.ingramcontent.com/pod-product-compliance
Lightning Source LLC
Chambersburg PA
CBHW072004070526
44583CB00015B/1329